Runner's World

INDOOR EXERCISE BOOK

Runner's World

INDOOR EXERCISE BOOK

**by Richard Benyo
and Rhonda Provost**

Runner's World Books

Library of Congress Cataloging in Publication Data

Benyo, Richard.
   Indoor exercise book.

   1. Physical fitness for women. 2. Exercise.
I. Provost, Rhonda, 1948-   joint author.
II.Title.

GV482.B38   613.7'045   80-39600
  ISBN 0-89037-190-3 (spiral)

Contents

Dedication. vi
Introduction I. vii
Introduction II xii
1.   Warm Bodies. 1
2.   No-Fuss Fitness. 29
3.   The Bucket Brigade. 55
4.   Light Work 79
5.   Your Most Important Ten Minutes 111
6.   Heavy Equipment. 129
Appendices–Progression and Measurement Table. 144
            Weekly Journal 150
            Selected Hardware. 156
Acknowledgments. 180
About the Authors 180
Recommended Reading. 181

Dedication

For our parents who, through their example, showed us that it's just as easy to go through life physically active as it is to grow moss—and who showed us that it can be twice the fun.

Introduction I

If all of us were born perfectly fit, we would not stay that way. Nature and circumstances have laid too many traps along life's road—traps that whittle away at the physical ideals that we can be.

Traps like aging. Like ice cream sundaes. Like jobs and kids and housework and overtime and TV and Pepperidge Farms layer cakes.

It would be fair to picture each of us as an ideal person wandering, like Dorothy, down a yellow-brick road. Only our road has potholes filled with chocolate syrup, overhanging trees filled with the fruits of frustration and stress, and detours on roads leading to nowhere that keep us occupied doing a lot of nothing while we grow older and more tired.

An obsession with getting ahead in life often leaves us precious little time or energy to enjoy that for which we've worked so hard. That striving for betterment is often the culprit. We often work like demons to get our little portions of heaven on earth, only to realize that we're too spent to reap its rewards.

I can remember the insipid fitness of youth. I'm sure you can, too. During high school, we could go at full-tilt each and every day, as though there were a nuclear power plant somewhere inside each of us. We were active and filled with energy. The only time we seemed to be running on empty was when there was some schoolwork or chores to be done.

For some of us, our energy levels had bad side effects. Unlike the brawny examples of youthful power and assertiveness in the Charles Atlas ads in the pages of comic books, many of us were downright skinny. "What's the matter with you?" my mother would say. "You eat like a horse and you still look like you've just come from a refugee camp." She was right; I ate like a horse. I don't know where the food was going, because after eating supper, both

my brother and I, because we liked what it tasted like and because
we wanted to get a bit of beef on us,would go to the local hang-
out and order slices of pizza and chocolate malts. The calories that
we ingested apparently escaped through our pores and into the air.
We remained embarrassingly skinny. "Aren't they giving you
enough to eat?" my grandmother would say when she saw me.
"Sure, sure they are," I'd say, moving imaginary sand around on
her kitchen floor with the toe of my right foot. As soon as she'd
get done giving her customary evaluation of my physique, I'd go
into her dining room and fill my pockets with the M & M's she
kept there for visiting marauders.

The tendency continued through college. I could eat four and
five times a day and never gain a pound. I had a part-time job at
the college cafeteria and would eat grapes and chocolate cake
while I swept the floors. Nothing.

What I didn't know was that all the calories you've eaten in
your youth get together in an alternate dimension and, when you
turn twenty-five (while you're trying to get settled in a job, a
lifestyle, trying to adjust to the real world, which often means
long hours and hard work and ignoring your body, which has
taken care of itself so well all these years), those calories begin
seeping through a rent in the fabric of the other dimension, and
they begin sneaking back into your body, hiding out in embarrassing places, such as the holsters of the lower rib-cage/upper hips.
They begin congregating there, waiting for the arrival of all their
friends from the other dimension, all of whom have been waiting
anxiously to make their appearance. Suddenly, the next time your
mother sees you, she begins saying things like: "My, you're finally
starting to fill out." Or your father says: "I'm glad to see he's
finally getting some beef on him."

As though adding weight were healthy.

Unfortunately, like most negative things in life, your misfortunes come in threes.

- you're adding weight
- you're losing muscle tone
- you're losing stamina

What it amounts to is very simple. You're *out of shape.*

Consider, for a moment, the negative response one gets from
the use of the words "out of."

"Gosh, here it is, 2:30 a.m., the middle of nowhere, and we're
out of gas."

"Well, Mr. Wabash, as your psychologist for seventeen years, I'm afraid that I've come to the conclusion that you're *out of* your mind."

"Yes, dear, I know you like your chocolate cake iced but it's a holiday, there are no stores open, and we're *out of* sugar."

"Yes, I know you've come a long way. But the mule teamsters are having their convention here in Bethlehem this year, and we're clean *out of* rooms at the inn."

"Yes, mirror, I see what you're saying. I'm only twenty-five years old, but I'm terribly *out of* shape."

Unfortunately, the out of shape monster seems to sneak up on us so fast that before we even know he's there with his army of calories storehoused in the other dimension for ten years, he has pushed the battle forward and we feel on the edge of defeat.

Life has so occupied us with diversionary tactics that the enemy has made a substantial beachhead before we ever realize we've been attacked. It is very frustrating to make the discovery that we're no longer in shape, that we are no longer even in neutral territory—we're just plain out of shape! Ugh.

Some people just give up the battle at that point, throwing up their hands in surrender. Some even sneak up to the enemy camp and go over to the other side, aggravating the problem by sitting around (inactively) worrying about it, sublimating their frustration (actively) by eating away that frustration, and waiting around (inactively) to develop ulcers, or else waiting to come to grips with the fact that all is lost, so you'd best make the best of it.

For some people, to mount an attack seems hopeless.

After all, little has been altered in their lifestyles. One honest look in the mirror at the perspiration that's accumulated on the forehead from trying to walk up the steps too fast, and at the extra pounds around the middle, does not alter the fact that you've still got to earn a living, or take care of the house and kids, or go on with a certain number of hours in the day dedicated to a set routine. It is not easy to find time, energy and motivation to break out of a routine that you've worked so hard to build over the years.

The problem is simply that we are allowing ourselves to be overwhelmed. We are still obsessed with the pictures in the Charles Atlas ad in the comic books. We are still obsessed with what we used to look like ten years ago, or fifteen years ago, and let's face it, even Charles Atlas no longer looks like he looked as a kid.

Can you picture him in his first grade class picture with all the buttons torn off his shirt because he flexed his mighty chest when the photographer said, "Okay, boys and girls, everybody straighten your back, make your mouths smile, and push out your chests."

Let's be realistic.

We aren't kids anymore. Thank God.

If someone were to come up to us and ask us what we want most in life, we aren't going to say, "I wanna be built like Charles Atlas." On a priority list of one hundred things we'd like, being built like Charles Atlas is probably not even in the running on our booby prize list of ten.

So why do we kid ourselves? Why do we frustrate ourselves by picturing someone like Charles Atlas when we say fit?

What we should mean when we say fit is three things:

1. My weight should be within acceptable limits for my height and age. (Translation: I should not look as though I escaped from the pachyderm tent at Ringling Bros., Barnum & Bailey Circus.)

2. My muscles and skin should not droop. (Translation: I should not look and feel as though I'm hiding inside a rubber suit that is four sizes too big for me.)

3. I should be able to go about daily activities, including walking several flights of steps, without having to stop to catch my breath. (Translation: I should not have to move through life with an oxygen tank strapped to my back.)

To be in shape, a person does not have to progress to the point where he or she can lift his or her body weight above the head, have muscles that can pop metal bands when flexed, or run a marathon every other week.

To be in shape, a person does not have to dedicate many hours a day to building bulky muscles, maintaining a specific weight level, and running or biking great distances. Some of those very concepts are in disagreement with each other. You don't see many world-class marathoners looking like the Incredible Hulk.

You can put yourself in shape in a reasonable, sane way, at home, with a minimum of time expended, with a minimum of fuss and hassle, and without making a big deal about it until you are ready to call attention to it. You don't have to wait until the dark of night to go out running so that no one can see you trying to run off twenty pounds; you don't have to work with massive weights and go to a gym where many of the people are going to be smoking while they're trying to get themselves in shape; you don't have to invest in a truckload of equipment; and, you can do it at your own speed, with your own goals in mind.

This book is not a guide to becoming musclebound and is not intended to build muscle bulk; to do that properly, you need an investment of a great deal of time at a gym, and just because one has bulky muscles does not necessarily mean the person is in shape. This book is not a guide to frustrating yourself with a great number of complex exercises.

This book is a layman's guide to controlling your weight, toning your muscles, and developing some degree of stamina. The book is meant to be light, irreverent, conversational, functional—it is certainly not the bible of fitness (it does not lay claim to being the *only* way to become fit at home), and is meant as only a starting point for a return to being in shape.

Hopefully, it will offer some logical, sensible ways of making fitness an integral part of your daily life. And it can fit in very easily with your other activities. I recommend that people who find it difficult to motivate themselves get together with friends and do the program jointly, as a social event. If you're a housewife who gets together for coffee a few mornings a week with friends, why not work some of these exercises into the sessions? If you and your partner do things at home as a couple, whether it be doing the bills once a week or watching television, you can do many of the exercises while sitting at the table or during the commercials. Some of the exercises can be done at breakfast, others you can do in bed.

I personally prefer to do exercising outdoors, whether it's running or bicycling. When I get home from a run though, I do a series of exercises on the living room floor while my muscles are still warmed up and more supple than they are before I exercise outdoors. (I have notoriously stiff and unyielding muscles.) I don't always do the exercises, unfortunately. But the next day, when I run or cycle again, my muscles remind me that I didn't do the exercises the day before. They don't want to cooperate because they haven't been trained to cooperate.

You'll be surprised how well your body responds, once it is trained to respond, once it is set in motion on a fitness program even if the program is of very modest means. There is an in shape person inside every one of us. It is all a matter of relativity. The most fit person you know probably has potential to be even more fit; that person, however, will have a tremendous amount of work before him or her to improve significantly. If you are currently what you consider out of shape, you have the potential for achieving greatness within and for yourself. Pull up a piece of wall or a chair and read this book. There is nothing in it that is impossible; some of the things are, in fact, fun. I'd suggest that you read the book through once, and then begin it over, starting your program at that point. You should do that to assure yourself that there are no trick endings, no chapters at the end that have you running the Pikes Peak Marathon or doing five thousand sit-ups.

The last chapter is an examination of the exercising equipment you can buy for your home. Equipment that, if you live in an apartment complex, will likely get you thrown out if you use it. You don't really have to read the final chapter if you want to keep this whole thing simple. There—see how easy it is? You've already saved some time and effort.

If there is a trick ending to this whole thing, it is twofold:

1. There is no ending; fitness should be an on-going thing.

2. When you're comfortable with yourself exercising indoors, if the weather calls you outside to continue your exercises, go to it. The world is your exercise yard; the privacy of your own home was merely the bullpen.

—Richard Benyo
Palo Alto, California
October 1980

Introduction II

My paternal grandfather succumbed to a bout of influenza when my father was two years old; his wife joined him a few short years later when one of the valves of her heart failed to function properly. My father, along with his brother and sister, were suddenly orphans.

My father has always led an exemplary life with regard to his physical well-being. I can't help but believe that the early deaths of both his parents convinced him that the hereditary factors in his life were not conducive to longevity.

Assuming that he had that strike against him, he went through life overcompensating in other areas. He was very active in his youth. Unlike many of us, he maintains that high level of activity to this day. He has never smoked, imbibes in the spirits only on a social basis, and as a result of sensible eating habits, weighs today what he weighed in high school. He is scheduled to retire in early 1981. (Let me add that both his brother and sister died, like their parents, at relatively young ages. While my father was getting in touch with and listening to his body, they were severely abusing theirs. It cost them their lives).

My father recently agreed to a very extensive physical, which I'd been suggesting for years. The results? It came as no surprise that he's in excellent health—as good as, if not better than, many men thirty years his junior. And all simply because he's been good to his body.

It gives me pleasure to see people like my father living healthy lives. I derive an equal amount of gratification from knowing that they refuse to fall victims to what so many of us do...inertia.

"Inertia!?" you might say.

"There aren't enough hours in my day to do all the running around I have to do. I get up early, then I....

a. feed the children and see them off to school

b. spend much of my day doing laundry and cleaning the house

c. rush out to work with hardly any time to eat

d. race around all day doing miscellaneous errands (i.e., food shopping, post office, etc.)

e. all of the above."

Those are the mechanics of daily living. We all need to do a certain amount of "running around" solely to exist. The inertia I'm referring to is that tendency we all have to be indisposed to physical or mental motion or change.

"Who has time or energy during or at the end of a typical day to move or exert themselves?" you may ask.

My father experienced the problems of living as we all do. Supporting and helping to raise his seven offspring occupied most of his time. He didn't have enough extra time or energy to run or bicycle long distances. He belonged to no tennis clubs, racquetball clubs, or health spas. Yet he always had an abundance of physical and mental energy.

As a child, I recall being fascinated at his ability to stand, feet together, in front of our large livingroom chair and to broad-jump over it. He'd land, feet still together, on the other side. My sisters and I loved it, so he'd perform the feat again and again for us. What a workout his arms and legs were getting!

He loves to swim. During the summers, he'd take advantage of the weather and go for very long swims in the bay near our home. And he was always walking and encouraging us to do the same.

As a young man, he'd leave for work every day with three sandwiches in his lunch bag. As he got older he was aware that his requirements for food were diminishing, so he cut down to two sandwiches. As he nears his retirement, he now goes to work carrying only one sandwich.

I suppose I could formulate quite a list of all those little things he has done in his life that have together contributed to the good health and fitness he enjoys today. But I guess it would all boil down to the same thing.

He practiced good health habits. He didn't sporadically embark on fad diets. He always ate slowly and sensibly. When traveling or at home, if he was tired, he slept. He got plenty of exercise doing the things he enjoyed (i.e., swimming, sports, etc.) when he could. But if weather or time didn't permit that, he didn't suffer for it because his fitness was an on-going process in the way he walked (briskly) or functioned (efficiently utilizing good body mechanics). Over a period of years, those things make a substantial difference.

Being healthy and fit is the condition of being sound in body and mind. It's not necessary to have extraordinary muscle strength or physical stamina to be healthy. And physical and mental fitness doesn't absolutely protect one from disease. But being fit in body can't help but spill over to your psychological well-being. The more you move, the more adrenalin is available in your body at any given time. Adrenalin is the substance in your body that is partially responsible for, among other things, your state of mind. Establishing a sound equilibrium between the mind and the body is the recipe to use to improve the quality of your life.

The body is a fascinating machine in many ways, one of which is its ability to adapt to widely varied situations. We adapt to our normal daily environment and to the activity required of us by developing our muscle strength and exercise stamina proportional to our daily physical demands. We can take everyday situations and use them to our advantage. And then we can try to supplement our good health habits with regular exercise of some sort, whether it be swimming, bicycling, running, racquetball, or the exercises outlined in this book.

The more we demand of our body, the more it will provide. And by subjecting your body to regular periods of positive stress (i.e., exercise of any sort), you render it better able to withstand negative stress: those tensions of the body and mind that threaten to alter the existent equilibrium we try to maintain. Let me hasten to add, however, that if left in a less-stressful environment, you will also adapt to the lessened demand. That, unfortunately, is where too many of us lie—in an inert posture. Don't use your daily routine as an excuse to avoid fitness. And don't underestimate your body. It's a fine, capable machine if you are patient and sensible and give it a chance.

This book approaches fitness from the same angle that my father, whether knowingly or unknowingly, approached it—as a natural part of his life. It's written on the premise that it shouldn't be something separate and apart from the rest of your life, to be thought about only when engaged in strenuous physical exercise. Instead of hindering your academic, personal, or occupational pursuits, fitness can and should be incorporated into them as part of a natural process to enhance your stamina with a resultant increase in your physical and mental well-being.

We understand that anyone, whether young or old, who has been inactive will have lost physical stamina and will become fatigued with minimal exertion; therefore, your readaptation to the stress of exercise may be slow. Bearing that in mind, we've presented the chapters so that they contain graded levels of exercise. We feel this is the way you should become reacquainted with your physical self. The book begins with the simple and progresses to the more complex. Factors such as motivation, ability, and practice will influence individual progress. We recommend reading through the book once before embarking on a serious program..

It's your body, and we hope you make a special attempt to get in touch with it and listen to it. Your body is the vehicle in which you travel through life. Maintain it.

—Rhonda Provost
Palo Alto, California
October 1980

1

Warm Bodies

A nut case resides in the apartment complex across the street. We don't know his name or what he looks like and we'd rather go through the rest of our lives in ignorance of those points. We're fearful that if we knew who he was, we'd have an urge, when seeing him on the street, to walk straight up to him, grab him by the throat and throttle him to within an inch (or less) of his life.

The guy, you see, commits assault upon our sensibilities in two ways:

1. He destroys our precious and well-earned sleep.

2. He mistreats dumb machinery.

What he does is inflict extreme torture to the engine of his car. He does so, once a week, at the ungodly hour of 5:45 a.m.

Our alarm clock is set for 6:00 a.m. It is set on a soothing radio station so that we are awakened gently to soft music. We then roll over, become aware of the fact that it is time to wake up, and catch the news so we can get an update on what is happening in the world outside before venturing out into something that we would have liked to be warned about. We get very little time to read the newspaper, so the update of world and local events is valuable. We would hate, for instance, to be waiting for a newspaper to tell us that during the night we'd suffered an atomic attack, when we can get the news from the radio in time to decide not to go to work that day. For people who must rise at 6:00 a.m., then, the half-hour before the radio wakes them is very treasured time.

Once a week, however, we are jerked from our sleep as the still of the morning air is rent by the sound of a car's starter grinding three floors below our open bedroom window. This particular car does not start very easily. The owner apparently does not know why it does not leap instantly to life; *we* know why it does not leap instantly to life: it's because the poor, miserable engine is on its last gasp before it self-destructs.

The guy sits there and grinds away at the engine. You can follow his mounting anger at the car's reluctance to start by the increasing number of tries he makes per minute. If we were the car, we'd just plum refuse to start. Period. Because when he finally coaxes, cajoles and beats the car into life, he proceeds to hold the accelerator to the floorboards so that the poor engine, that has spent all night in the cool air, is suddenly reviving itself at about 7000 rpms. The poor little engine sounds like a cat with a dump-truck parked on its tail. It screams like a banshee.

It becomes, naturally enough, very difficult to continue a sound sleep when a wall of sound is assailing you from outside your window. It is a doubly painful awakening because we know what the poor engine is going through.

When a car's engine sits all night, two things happen to the oil, the engine's lifeblood. One thing is that it drips to the bottom of the engine, way down into the oilpan. The other thing is that as it cools, it thickens, until it becomes the consistency of molasses. When the engine is fired up, then, the parts in the upper portion of the engine (these are the more delicate parts, and the majority of the engine's moving parts) have no oil on them, so they are rubbing against each other while dry. Run a knife down a dinner plate. You get the idea. Those parts are hoping for a quick shot of oil so they'll be lubricated against that painful friction. They will eventually get oil, as it's pumped from the bottom of the engine and sprayed over the moving parts. But it takes a few moments for that to happen. That's why engines are built with certain mechanisms on the choke that regulate the rpms the engine endures during those first important moments. That's why it is wise to give the engine a few moments, before engaging the clutch or automatic transmission, to properly oil itself—gently.

When one revs the engine from the instant that it comes to life, there is a great rasping of metal against metal, and there is a very rapid building of friction—and with friction, comes heat. By the time the oil is pumped up to the top of the engine, there is already metal worn off—metal that the oil then washes through the engine. Picture the effect on your stomach of swallowing a handful of iron filings.

So this poor little engine is held to maximum revs for about two minutes, the driver apparently figuring he's doing two things:

1. Recharging his battery, which may have lost some juice while he tried unsuccessfully to start the car.

2. Teaching the engine a lesson—punishing it, so to speak, for not jumping to life at the first turn of the key.

(Unfortunately, like an infant with diarrhea, spanking it only makes the situation more acute.)

The engine, then, is suffering for something over which it has no control. And the punishment is aggravating the problem.

Automobile engines don't function properly until they are given a chance to warm up—gently.

It is very similar with the human body. We sometimes grind our teeth when we see people walk right out the door first thing in the morning to take off on a run, without giving their bodies the least bit of a chance to warm-up. They go off at a vigorous pace and, fifteen minutes later, come staggering back, looking worse than death warmed over.

The human body functions best when it is warmed up and the parts can move easier; it functions best when it is not put to extreme usage right away, while it is still relatively cold. Even once warmed up, it needs to be eased into exercise and activity. Watch the incredibly slow warm-up laps that a NASCAR Grand National stock car is given before it is brought up to speed.

For someone who wants to become active following a serious period of non-use, the best way to start is to *not* start. Seriously. No matter how much you want to get into an ambitious exercise program, no matter how much you want to tighten up the thighs, tone the arms, and build stamina, *don't rush into it.*

Perhaps the major shortcoming of Americans is that they are impatient people. "If we can fly from coast to coast in five hours, why can't I become fit in five weeks...?"

We see talented people who take up a sport like running end up on the sidelines, watching other people do what they could have done better, simply because they tried to do it all at once. Instead of building a foundation, then the first story, and so forth, they tried to build the peak (attic) of their fitness in thin air. You can imagine the pile of rubble that resulted.

Patience, then, is the key word. Fitness through exercise is a lifetime commitment, not a one-night rendezvous.

Just as the guy with the poor little car should have been patient with it, should have let it warm at its own speed, so you should ignore the urge to go fast. Anyone who tells you that they are going to make you healthy and fit in an incredibly short period of time should be made to lie under this guy's engine next time he starts it on a cold morning.

The body, like the engine, has parts that move against each other. When those parts are cold, and when they are not lubricated, they tend to grate—and grating causes friction, and friction causes damage. What the car's motor has going for it is that if some parts are worn badly, they can be replaced by parts that are waiting on a service station's shelf. If you wear down a joint or a bone, or tear into a muscle, your body has some of its own service station-like functions that can repair it, but if it's too serious, it isn't going to heal—and even if it heals, it isn't like it's a fresh, new, unused part.

So how should you start?

You should begin by intimately learning your body's needs in the warm-up phase. In fact, you could learn the warm-up phase as an entity unto itself. A warm body functions better than a cold body. If you go no farther in this book than learning how to warm up your body properly, you are doing yourself—and it—a great service. (And, on some days, with your schedule being what it is, you may not have enough time to do a complete series of exercises. But on almost any day, you have enough time to warm up the body so that it moves through the day with a great deal more ease and efficiency).

Let's just refer to this whole phase as warm-up. It is a combination of many disciplines (including yoga, stretching, calisthenics, etc.) that have been customized into something much simpler and easier to handle. Some people are turned off by the very thought of yoga; it conjures up visions of lonely people in India sitting on top of mountains looking very forlorn as they are bent into a shape resembling a pretzel while gazing off into space as though in a semi-coma. Stretching, on the other hand, has mixed response: one either thinks of the Spanish Inquisition or of luxuriously stretching before getting out of bed on a languid Sunday morning before the life outside your bedroom interrupts. Calisthenics. Well, we all remember boring gym classes where we had to do jumping jacks and toe-touches and sit-ups, looking much like an army trying to collectively end a siege of constipation.

Warm-ups should be pleasurable and painless and should conjure up images of lazy Sunday mornings just before getting out of bed, cats going through their stretching maneuvers just as they get up from a good nap, and a quiet beach of white silvery sand with a warm sun beating down caressingly on your muscles, making them warm and loose and supple.

The sequence of warm-ups in this chapter can very easily be done as a part of waking up. You can be warmed up before ever leaving your bedroom in the morning. Or you can do them at various points during the day when you feel tense and you have a few moments to yourself when you can get loose without working up a sweat.

We'll go over these simple warm-ups leisurely, which is how all exercise should be approached. Approach everything in this book at—remembering the automobile engine—an idle. Don't rush it, don't rev the engine. If you have to rush it, either don't do it or put it off until tomorrow; it's better to not do it than to hurt yourself trying to rush it. To rush it is to do it wrong; to rush it is definitely to do it inefficiently and gratingly; and often, to rush it is to rush past many of the benefits. And sometimes to rush into injury from something that was supposed to be beneficial.

Besides tightening up your muscles in a positive way, these exercises should also loosen up your tensions.

So let's get started—gently.

We'll look briefly at your body machine and then we'll get into the warm-ups. You don't need any special equipment. The only clothing you need is something comfortable that will flex with you—or nothing at all, which flexes best.

THE BASIC BODY MACHINE

The body is the most wonderful organic machine we know. Perhaps someday, we (as a race) will encounter another race of beings with more sophisticated organic systems than ours. But at the moment, your body is the most sophisticated organic machine anyone has discovered. It is more intricate than the most complex computer, with functions going on at a cellular level that are controlled by small recesses in our brains, but that never have to consciously be thought about as long as we live. The functions are on auto-pilot; when we need them they are there to adjust our bodies to its environment and to the stresses being put on it. Unlike a man-made machine, our bodies still hold many of their secrets intact; as long as man has known his body, he has never come to fully understand it—and probably never will.

Using the analogy of the automobile, consider the amazement we would all exhibit if the Ford Motor Company unveiled a new car that did everything without being told. A car that started automatically, that turned on its lights when needed, that drove its owner wherever he or she wanted to go, that was constantly repairing itself, that was constantly shedding its paint job (on a microscopic level) to expose bright, new paint. Consider the amazement a car would cause that could potentially run for seventy-five years with minimum maintenance.

Exercise places demands on all the individual systems that collectively comprise the body machine. The conscious and unconscious mechanisms in the brain bring muscle, heart, lung and other systems into play during exercise, with each system being very much interrelated.

Most of us approach exercise for reasons other than the mere pleasure of movement and putting the body to work. We hope to lose a few pounds or a few inches so we can feel and look better. Once the exercise routine has become a regular part of a person's day, however, it becomes doubly interesting to begin to learn the inner workings of the body during exercise phases. What determines energy and fatigue levels? Why is it seemingly easier to exercise on some days than on others? Why do I sweat when exercising? Why do I sweat more when I stop exercising than I did while I was actually performing the exercise? Why does exercising make me breathe harder and faster? Why, the day or two following exercise, do I feel sore, while on other days I don't seem to mind it? When should I eat relative to when I exercise? Does eating make exercise more difficult?

We'll take a few moments to examine the functioning of the body machine before starting its motor to do warm-ups.

The primary event in exercising is muscle contraction, with all other systems playing a supporting role. To exercise, in other words, you must move, and movement is done by the muscles.

The chief fuel source for active muscles is glycogen, which is stored in the muscles and the liver. The body calls upon this energy source when it embarks on either aerobic or anaerobic activity. (Aerobic means in the presence of oxygen, while anaerobic means in the absence of oxygen. Aerobic exercise would be any sustained exercise that does not cause the person to begin gasping for air; anaerobic exercise occurs when you begin gasping for more air than you are able to ingest with normal breathing, i.e., if you sprint as opposed to jog.)

Exercising at the aerobic level makes use of a mix of oxygen being taken into the body with energy sources already in the body in the form of fats, proteins and carbohydrates. The oxygen is needed to help produce the energy, just as air must be taken in through a car's carburetor, where it is mixed with gasoline and ignited, in order to convert fuel to energy.

Hold your hand in front of your face. Flex the fingers. That simple movement consumed a small amount of fuel in your body, while the body pulled in just a mite more oxygen than it would have at rest to turn the fuel to energy. That movement of the fingers of your hand did several things: it instigated the use of energy within your body, produced heat in the burning of the fuel, and produced a small amount of waste by-product (in the form of lactic acid). Just like a car. Start the engine and move it a foot forward. The engine burns fuel, begins to warm and blows exhaust out the muffler. In both the example of the human hand and the mechanical car, oxygen was necessary to burn the fuel.

Unlike the car, though, the muscle can function without immediately available oxygen—but for a very limited time. This happens in anaerobic exercise. The energy for the flexing of the muscle, in that case, comes directly from the glycogen stores in the liver or within the muscle. The body has trouble dissipating the heat and the waste products fast enough during anaerobic exercise.

In strenuous exercise, muscle fatigue is due in part to exhausting muscle glycogen stores. Residual lactic acid and muscle fatigue brought about from them being unused to such activity can combine to cause initial soreness. The object of turning the body into a more efficient machine is to turn what was anaerobic and unusual activity into aerobic and normal activity. In other words, what you'll be able to do six months from now will make what you have trouble doing now seem absurd.

Don't let some muscle soreness discourage you. Again using the analogy of the warmed engine, once you begin moving again, much of the soreness disappears. The soreness is a positive indicator that you have been doing something to raise your body's effectiveness to a new level. This tendency toward soreness will diminish as you become stronger and more used to the exercise. By starting slowly, you will be assisting your body in keeping up with disposing of the waste materials; they will be pumped out of your system with the massaging action of muscular movement.

The increased metabolism associated with exercise results in increased body temperature. (An engine being run at 5000 rpms produces more heat than one running at 1200 rpms.) One of the body's methods of maintaining a body temperature that is tolerable to all body systems is sweating. By covering itself with a film of moisture, the body provides heat loss by evaporation. The air surrounding the body evaporates the sweat, and with the evaporation, heat is dissipated. In order to bring blood close enough to the surface of the skin so that sweating may occur, large amounts of blood are diverted from the active muscles that need it. As a result, sweating occurs in the most copious amounts after you've completed your exercises and your muscles can afford to let the blood be shunted to the skin. A similar process occurs when exercising on a full stomach; blood is diverted to the stomach to aid in digestion, and is then not available to help deal with the needs of the exercising muscles, causing the muscles to become fatigued more easily.

A word of caution: When exercising, with all of these body systems operating, try to avoid being interrupted, whether it's by chatting on the phone or watching your favorite television program. To interrupt your exercise is to signal your systems to begin shutting down; when you restart, therefore, your tendency will be to begin where you left off, whereas your body has returned to the level it was before you started your exercise routine, and should be again eased into full functioning. To jump right back into your exercise program after an interruption is to chance muscle pulls and stiffness, and it may cause unnecessary fatigue by forcing your body to rapidly catch up to you again.

The role of the lungs in exercise is threefold: they provide needed oxygen, aid in the removal of waste products, and aid in the removal of excess heat.

Much of the lactic acid we spoke of before as a by-product of exercise can be broken down within the body and excreted, in another form, through the breath; the increased breathing that accompanies exercise brings in extra oxygen while exhaling waste gasses.

Following exercise, the breathing will return gradually to normal. At that point, the lactic acid and other liquid waste products remaining in the body begin the slow process of finding their own way out of the muscles, and from there out of the body, usually through urination.

One question about breathing that seems to be raised frequently among people new to exercise is this: "When I exercise, should I breathe through my nose or my mouth?" The answer is to do whatever it takes; if you are exercising slowly and easily and breathing through your nose is enough, that's fine; if you find you need more air, breathe through the mouth also. You'll take in much more oxygen while ridding yourself of much more waste. Again, remember the automobile. The larger the carburetor, the more air is taken in to the combustion chamber and the more energy is released; the larger the exhaust pipe, the more volume of waste gas can be expelled.

While you are breathing harder to match your increasing workload, your body is sending more blood to your lungs in order to pick up and distribute the increased air supply. It's all happening automatically, your body functioning like the advanced machine it is. If you find yourself straining a bit with your breathing, take two or three deep breaths between warm-ups or exercises. Just don't spend too much time taking breaths between each exercise, or you'll begin to allow the body to cool down. By moving on to the next warm-up or exercise briskly you can more closely approach ideal aerobic exercise, which will exercise your heart and blood vessels as well as your muscles. Sustained exercise, as long as it does not strain you, is the most beneficial.

By exercising at a steady rate, the heart and blood vessels are exercised, the heart by pumping blood faster and by getting a work-out in the process, and the vessels by expanding to accommodate the increased blood flow that exercising requires.

The massaging action of the muscles during exercise also aids blood in returning to the heart. The blood passes through the lungs, and exchanges waste products for a new supply of oxygen, and then returns to the heart to be pumped to all organs. All in all, a most ingenious system, and one that would be worth copying in some of mankind's machines.

Armed with a better appreciation of what will happen when you put your body into a warm-up and ultimately an exercise routine, let's briefly discuss the all-important topic of motivation. If the body is such a marvelous machine and functions so wonderfully, why make it do more than it is doing? And, if I decide that I want it to do more, how do I convince myself that I should do it regularly? Good questions that deserve good answers.

THE CRITICAL QUESTION: "WHY BOTHER?"

All things in life can be defined in a very structured manner. Let's try constructing a very structured definition for exercising:

Exercise is a psychological and physical event beginning with the knowledge that there is a task to be performed. After coordination of all body systems in order to execute the task, exercise concludes with satisfaction or relief that the task has been completed.

This is rather a structured way of saying: Decide that you want to do it. Tell your body that you want it to do it. Get it done. Sit back and enjoy the results.

It sounds very, very easy. Actually, it is. All a person needs is the motivation to do it. There is apparently a good foundation of motivation present in you to embark on an indoor exercise program, or you wouldn't be reading this book. There are probably as many reasons for becoming motivated to start an exercise program as there are people doing it. But let's take a look at some possible motivators and see if any of them strike a responsive chord:

1. A desire for improved muscle tone. Doing away with a few excess inches that have creeped up when you weren't looking can generate plenty of positive feedback from family and friends, and can be quite evident when you meet yourself each morning in front of the mirror. Exercising doesn't always promise that a person will *lose pounds,* but it almost always adjusts the pounds into a more favorable presentation. One drawback: You'll have to alter many of your clothes, or perhaps purchase some new ones.

2. Loss of weight. The increase in metabolism that accompanies *regular* exercise persists not only while you're exercising but extends much of a twenty-four hour period. Therefore, calories are utilized at a consistently higher rate.

3. Higher energy levels, lower fatigue. In a stressful situation (and exercise is a *positive* stress situation), certain body hormones are called into play. One of these hormones is adrenalin. As a result of the release of this substance into the system (which, recall, has effects that last nearly a day), the activity and excitability of the whole body is increased. This increase results in higher energy levels and therefore less fatigue.

4. The challenge. For people who enjoy the challenges in life, to get into shape and to stay there is an ongoing challenge that may be somewhat low-key in comparison to challenges like climbing high mountains and holding one's breath underwater for a record time, but that is certainly worthy of the mettle of any man or woman.

5. Increased strength, endurance and/or efficiency. Exercise trains the body to perform its daily tasks with a decreased amount of energy; in other words, when you're in shape, you have the option of either doing what you do with less energy used, or expending the same amount of energy but accomplishing more. Over a period of time, you will begin increasing the energy stores available to you, so that, should a stressful or unexpected situation arise requiring plenty of extra energy, it will be there for your use.

6. Improved capacity to enjoy life. People who fall asleep at the slightest opportunity miss out on a lot in life. One thing they miss out on is a full sex life. If you exercise regularly and improve your strength, endurance and efficiency of body movements, there is no guarantee that your sexual technique will be improved, but it will certainly provide the means of practicing at those techniques more frequently.

7. Improved self-esteem. Setting goals of exercising regularly and meeting those goals does much to elevate self-esteem in a job well done. The exercise also has other side-effects that help self-esteem besides meeting goals, however. The adjustment in pounds and inches, and the feeling of power and strength within your body is bound to improve your self-esteem. To exercise is to have regard for yourself and for the vehicle that is you. To be successful in exercising and in making your body machine the best it can be is guaranteed self-esteem.

8. A desire to return. Perhaps you were a regular exerciser at one point in your life, but you allowed other things to throw you off the track. Recall how good you felt when you were exercising regularly. Welcome back!

BEFORE THE WARM-UP

Whatever your motivation for exercising, the process can't help but leave you with an increased overall sense of well-being and increased energy levels, all of which combine to improve your quality of life, something we took for granted when we were children, but something that becomes more precious as we become old enough to appreciate its far-reaching implications.

Before taking the great step into vigorous exercise, the proper warm-up is necessary, as we've already discussed. A proper warm-up is preventive maintenance for the body machine and even the most expert exerciser uses the warm-up as an integral part of the routine.

There are three things that *must* be stressed in warming-up:

1. Be patient. No matter what your level of fitness was during your youth, and no matter what level it is now, you must begin any new program *slowly*. A year from now, with hundreds of hours of exercise showing its benefits above your belt, you should still begin slowly. The human machine never adapts to going from a state of inactivity to activity without some sort of preparation. Don't spring surprises on your body; to do so is asking for trouble. If you jump from inactivity to activity without a warm-up, you are asking to jump into injuries. In doing any warm-up or exercise, proceed to the point of discomfort and no further. If you proceed too rapidly you'll push beyond that fine line before you know it, and you'll stress or strain yourself unnecessarily. As your body becomes used to this new daily routine, it'll adapt and your abilities will improve.

If your body is what you consider to be out-of-shape, it didn't get to be that way overnight; don't expect it to make a complete about-face in no time at all.

2. Be gentle. Let your mind as well as your body adjust to what you're demanding of it. Allow yourself the time to do the warm-ups and exercises. Don't push yourself mercilessly. If anything, the warm-ups should be very passive and very gentle. There will be plenty of opportunity for you to exert yourself once you move into the exercising. By being gentle with your body machine at this point, you will insure its limberness and willingness and ability to perform at its top efficiency later. Remember, this is the oiling process for the machine's engine; don't race the motor.

3. Relax. That's right, relax. With a capital "R". All good exertion is done in a relaxed, in-control manner. Watch a world-class marathoner run; he is performing at peak efficiency, but he is doing so because he is relaxed. Tension is like trying to drive efficiently while leaving the hand-brake engaged. Muscles and minds that are relaxed always function better than those under stress and duress. You'll be amazed at how frequently it is possible to become tense while going through the warm-up phase without even realizing it. Become aware from the start of the parts of your body that are tensing up in anticipation of the warm-up. Remember that the way you do your warm-ups are *your* way. You do not have to imitate someone else. Your body is unique. Enjoy the sensations that the warm-ups instigate; be aware of what your muscles are doing during warm-up. And Relax!

Armed with an appreciation of what the warm-up does for a cold body, and fortified by your own motivation, let's consider the matter of *when* you might want to do a warm-up sequence.

Whether doing warm-ups for themselves, or as preparation for doing a series of exercises, you should be aware that anything you do first thing in the morning will be done with a body that is probably as stiff as it's going to be at any point throughout the day, due specifically to its night of inactivity. Go about your morning warm-ups at a pace that is maddeningly slow. This will slowly bring up your circulation and will prepare you for what's ahead, whether it be a full set of exercises or a hard day around the house or at the office.

If it seems difficult to get the body moving first thing in the morning, a warm shower will serve to loosen up the limbs and create flexibility before you proceed to move under your own power. The shower should also help to clear your head after a good night's sleep.

Hopefully, you will plan on doing the warm-ups prior to eating. Doing virtually anything physical on a full stomach is asking for discomfort. Besides the needed blood being diverted to the stomach to process food as we've already discussed, exercising on a full stomach can cause stomach upset, cramps and premature fatigue.

You'll find very quickly that each of the ten warm-ups are easy and relaxing. You may want to occasionally work one or the other into your normal day when appropriate, when no one is around, or when the urge to feel good overtakes you after a few hours of inactivity at one job or the other. You do not have to be at a gym or in the privacy of your own home to do most of these without gathering a crowd. It's fun to sneak some of them in to keep your body loose and supple as the day wears on.

THE WARM-UPS

I. Just Hang Loose—Stand in the center of the room with your legs spread approximately two feet apart at the base, feet parallel. With your legs kept straight, bend at the waist and just let the arms hand toward the floor. Just let them hang loose; let gravity do the work. You'll be a bit tight initially, especially in the back of the thighs (hamstrings) and in the lower back. If you're doing this one first thing in the morning, you may find that there won't be much bending going on at the waist, but remember...be patient. Let gravity do the work for you. With fingers outstretched, just relax and over a period of about two minutes you should find that without straining, your muscles will passively stretch. Do this on a regular basis (as often as you feel comfortable doing it during the day) and you'll find that over a period of time your muscles will stretch to the point where you're able to place the palms of your hands flat on the floor! It has taken one of us years to master that little trick and there are still mornings when it is difficult to bend at the waist after a good night's sleep. But knowing one's body better now by making fuller use of it indicates that with patience it works. Give it a couple of minutes; just hang there; things will loosen up and stretch. (By the way, the other one of us still cannot do this one properly, so don't feel discouraged if your hands aren't on the floor the first day. Guess which one of us hasn't mastered it...)

Just Hang Loose

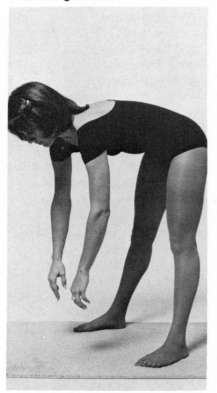 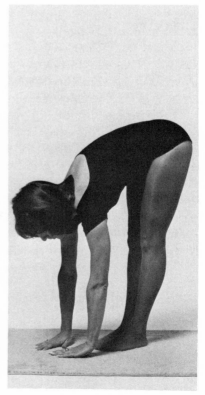

Do not begin by forcing your hands to the floor — let them fall toward it.

As you practice this one, you will eventually be able to palm the floor.

When you've mastered this with your legs spread, you might try bringing your feet together and once again hanging loose, keeping your legs straight. You're not going to be able to get as far as you were before, but don't get discouraged and *don't strain* to reach the floor. That's not the object of this maneuver; the object is again to work on it over a long period of time; if you don't master it today, there's always tomorrow.

II. Do Pull My Leg—Facing a wall, stand with your feet about three of your foot-lengths from the wall. Place your palms flat on the wall in front of you. Keep legs straight, heels and feet flat on floor and lean into the wall, bending at the elbows. Hold for five to ten seconds. Repeat three to five times. Maintain this position and flex the left leg while again leaning into the wall on the right leg. Return to the starting position, flex the right leg and lean into the wall on the left leg. This enables you to stretch your calf muscles and Achilles tendon (at the base of the calf, running down to the back of the heel) to a greater degree. Again, do this three to five times for five to ten seconds each time. This is also a good way to build strength in your upper arms.

Another good method of warming up and stretching your calves is to use a flight of stairs. Place the toes of both feet at the edge of the step while supporting yourself with your arms on the bannister. Hang off the edge of the step with your legs straight, allowing the heels to dip. Feel the muscles tighten in the back of your legs. Don't force them; again, let gravity do the work for you, and when they reach the point of discomfort, stop. Try to hold the stretch for five to ten seconds. Repeat it three times. A slight variation again involves the flexing and removing of weight from one leg while stretching the opposite, as you did against the wall. Then do the same on the other leg. This enables your muscles to passively stretch a little farther.

III. Cat Stretch—Kneel on the floor. Drop to all fours with your hands and knees spread about a foot apart, keeping them directly under you. Keep your back straight and your head up to look straight ahead. As you take a deep breath, arch your back up (as a cat does when it's angry) while simultaneously drawing your head down as far as you can, toward your chest. Hold and count slowly to three. Now, as you slowly exhale, let your back sink as far in as it will go without forcing it and simultaneously elevate your head. Again, hold to the count of three. Perform this set five times to loosen back muscles.

Do Pull My Leg

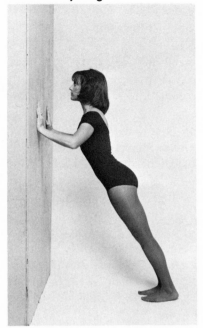 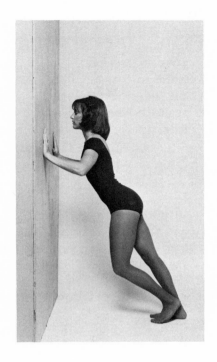

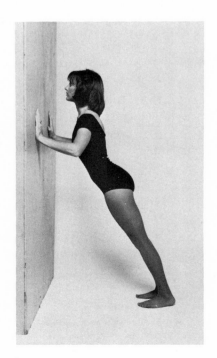

Several important points on this one: keep your legs straight when doing the exercise; use your arms to adjust your attitude to the wall to a comfortable level; concentrate on keeping your heels planted flat on the floor; don't hold the stretch too long (only to a count of 4 the first time, 6 the second time, 8 the third time); and pay attention to the places on the back of your leg where the stretching is occurring, being careful not to push it into the pain range.

Do Pull My Leg (cont'd)

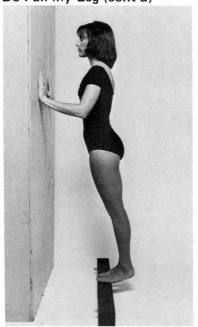

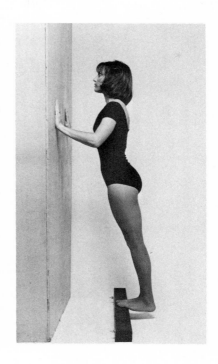

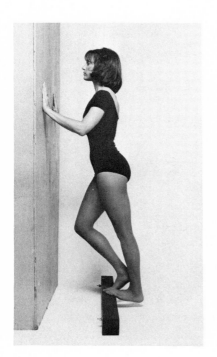

When doing this stretch on a step or a board, rest your toes on the edge, just near the balls of the foot (or about 40% back, where your foot flexes). If you do it while barefooted, be careful the board or step does not cut into the bottom of your foot. Do this much as you did the previous sequence, but do not rely so heavily on leaning into the wall; in this one, the wall is merely for support, while the controlled stress comes from your weight being pressed down upon your foot by gravity.

Cat Stretch

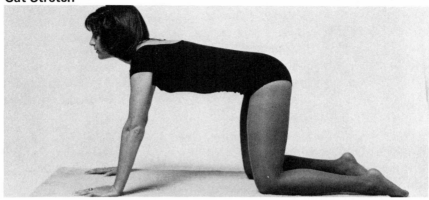

Form your body into a basic table, with back, arms and thighs straight.

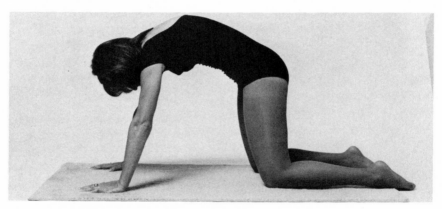

Arch your back toward the ceiling, like a cat coming out of a nap.

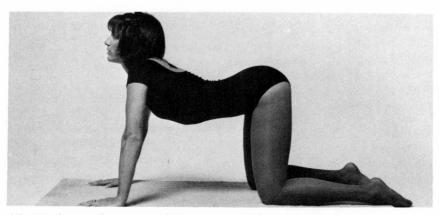

Allow gravity to pull your stomach down toward the floor, curving your back.

IV. The Twist—No, this isn't the one that Hank Ballard and the Midnighters first broke on the world, later to be made popular by Chubby Checker. This one is much easier. With your feet spread about two feet apart, hold arms straight out to the sides, parallel to the floor. Looking straight ahead, twist at the waist to simultaneously bring your right arm to the front of the body and the left arm back. Reverse. In one sweeping motion, bring the left arm to the front of the body while bringing the right arm to the back. This entire motion is done on a count of one. Be gentle but don't pause once started. With head still aimed forward, continue to do ten of these sequences. Remember, relax—keep your arms and legs straight.

V. The Rocking Chair—Maintain the same position as in number IV, with feet spread at the base and arms held out to the side, parallel to the floor. Looking straight ahead, bend at the waist to bring the left hand to the left knee while raising the right arm above the head. Return to the starting position. Then, bring the right hand to the right knee while raising the left arm above the head. This should all be done in a smooth, gentle, back-and-forth rocking fashion. Remember to keep your arms and legs straight.

VI. The Bob—Begin with your feet apart about two feet, arms extended to the sides as in IV and V. Bend forward at the waist and bob four times; then stretch to the left side with the right hand up, bobbing four times; lean back in slightly squat position, bobbing four times toward the wall behind you; stretch right, bob four times. Repeat this warm-up three times. Then, bob three times to each side; repeat it three times. Pause a moment, do two more sets of two to the sides, pause again and do one more set of two to each side.

VII. Running in Place—Now that your body has been stretched out a bit and has a little better idea of what you're demanding of it, take time to run in place gently for at least a minute, remembering to keep those thighs pumping high. If it's been a while since you've exercised, you'll be surprised how long a minute can be; if you have trouble lasting for a minute, don't push it to the point of great discomfort. This warm-up serves as an excellent means to get your heart beating faster and open up those vessels to your muscles to increase their blood supply. Again, begin this warm-up slowly, especially if you are coming off a long physical layoff. If you have a full-length mirror, do your running in place in front of it. Keep your arms relaxed and your body straight. Given

The Twist

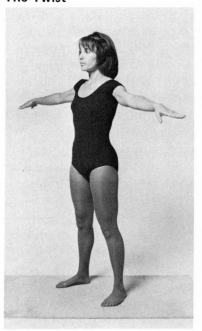

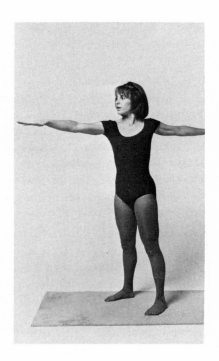

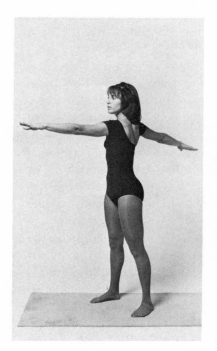

This one is very, very simple. The difficulty comes in keeping everything straight. The back should be perfectly vertical, the arms should be held straight, the legs should be straight. All rotation should come from the waist, almost as though you were automated, and everything were solid metal except for a single swivel joing in your midsection. Make your turn to the edge of comfort toward each side.

Rocking Chair

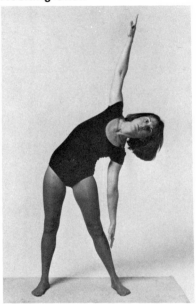 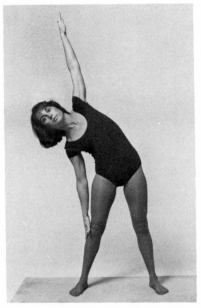

Again, the secret is to keep everything straight, especially the arms and legs.

Allow your fingers to just lightly brush your leg on each count; stay relaxed.

The Bob

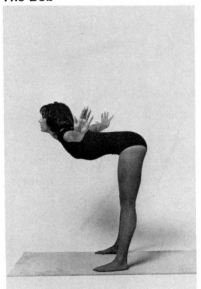 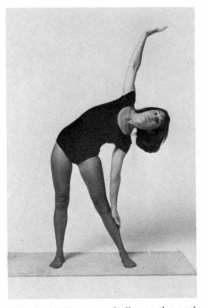

Keep your legs straight and control your bob forward with your toes dug into the rug.

This should be very similar to the position you were in with the Rocking Chair.

The Bob (cont'd)

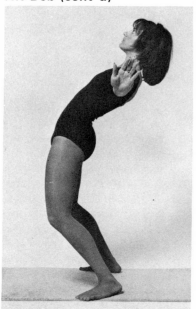

Do not bend back so far that you begin to cause pain in the lower back.

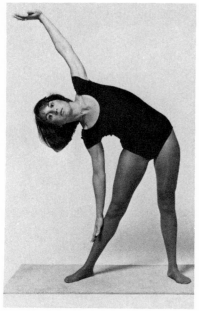

As you get better at this, you can touch your fingers even farther down your leg.

Running in Place

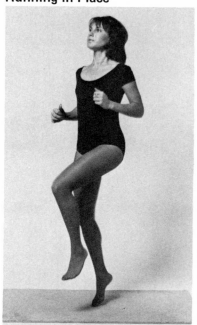

There are various pieces of hardware available to make this easier on the legs (including some equipment that looks very much like a small trampoline), but it can be done just as easily on a carpet or rug (making sure the rug does not slide out from under you). Do not exhaust yourself on this one; start your running very slowly, just a mere jog, and then, as you get better and warmer and stronger, you can lift your legs higher.

time, your strength and endurance will increase.

After this one, you'll likely want to stop for a moment and take a deep breath; take it slowly and enjoy it; don't pause beyond five good, deep breaths, though, as you want to keep your muscles warm.

VIII. Jumping Jacks—Here's one we all remember from high school phys ed class. If you didn't get to do them in high school, you've seen them on television or in the movies or on the football field where the players perform their pre-game warm-up exercises.

Begin by standing at attention, with your feet together and arms at your sides. On the count of one, jump, landing with your feet spread about two feet apart, while simultaneously clapping your hands over your head; jump again, returning to the at-attention position. This is a very easy one, once you've managed to coordinate both movements as you take off on the jump. Repeat the exercise ten times.

IX. Back Hand Clap—With your feet spread about two feet apart for a firm base, make loose fists with your hands. Join the knuckles of your fists in front of your chest, keeping the arms parallel to the floor. Now, push your elbows back, still keeping the arms parallel to the floor. Push them back twice. You should feel pulling in your chest and shoulders. On the third count, push your elbows toward the back again, but instead of keeping your fists forward, let your forearms swing with the backward movement, allowing your hands to clap behind your back. So it's two counts of pushing the elbows back, with your fists still aiming forward, followed by a hand-clap behind your back, followed by returning to your starting position. Repeat this one six times.

X. Great and Small Circles—Keep your feet spread apart and stretch your arms out to the sides, parallel to the floor. With the arms straight and the fingers together, use your arms to make ten small and vigorous circles forward; then reverse and do them backwards. Now, do ten large circles forward with your arms straight; and then do ten backwards.

Now, take a deep breath and relax. You've done the warm-up phase.

AFTER THE WARM-UPS

Remember that, at first, you'll experience some soreness. You'll also experience some soreness whenever you move to new exercises or increase the number or frequency of the exercises that you are already doing. Don't let that deter you. If you don't ex-

Back Hand Clap

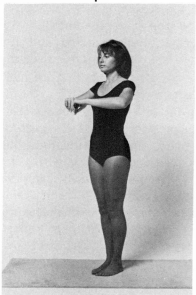

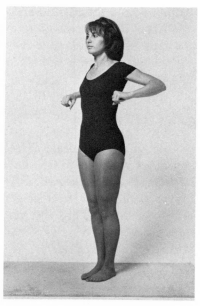

Stand straight, keeping your shoulders square and use only your arms.

Swing your arms back as though you were going to lean against the wall with your elbows.

Circles

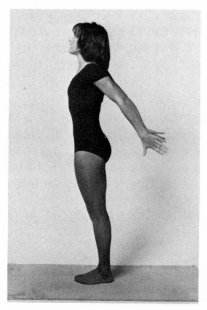

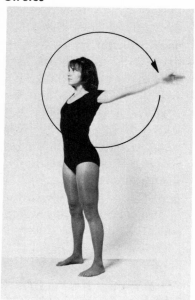

Clap your hands behind your behind; the clap does not have to be very hard.

Keep your body straight and only use the arms, swinging them freely.

perience some soreness, you probably aren't doing enough; it is a nice little way your body has of assuring you that something constructive is happening. It's similar to the signs you see at construction work on highways: *Temporary Inconvenience, Permanent Improvement.*

Even people who've been exercising for years can experience aches and pains and soreness—and often do. If you let your exercise slide for a bit (perhaps while you're on vacation, although that would seem like a perfect time to increase it), you'll feel some renewed soreness when returning to your regular exercise routine. (Rhonda here: I run more than twenty miles a week and bicycle extensively with a considerable expenditure of energy. As I sit here typing up the notes on this chapter, I am experiencing some discomfort when I sneeze—we just moved new bookcases in this afternoon and there is household dust in the air—and I'm stiff when I get up from the typewriter because two days ago I did the most extensive workout I've attempted in several weeks. And I'm almost perpetually active physically. You should see Rich after a twenty mile workout....! Or, worse yet, after an extensive session of stretching exercises. He's usually about as flexible as a piece of glass.)

Some of the things we find useful in minimizing soreness are:

1. Believe it or don't, continued activity! We try not to push our bodies too much, but occasionally we do overdo it. We suffer stiffness, usually the following day or two, and find that a bit of the hair of the dog, or more activity, will usually lessen the discomfort. It can be very uncomfortable at first, but after a few minutes, it really begins to work wonders. Just don't begin to feel so good that you again overdo it. The activity helps your body flush the lactic acid and other waste products from your body.

2. Drink plenty of fluids when you are exercising. Not while you are doing them, certainly, but right after you finish. Liquids are lost during exercise through sweating, and your body needs the fluids replaced. Fluids help maintain your chemical balance. Water is still the best all-around fluid you can use.

3. If you have a particularly sore spot on your body (your calf, perhaps), rubbing an ice cube on it after exercising will usually help it come back in no time. Don't put heat onto the sore muscle immediately after exercising, because the heat can cause swelling which will merely complicate the problem. If it's a choice between ice and heat, go with the ice. That will keep down the swelling and discomfort.

4. Soaking in a hot tub after icing the sore part of the body can be very relaxing, and since you've already prevented swelling with the ice, the heat will then have an opportunity to encourage increased blood supply to the injured area, thereby promoting the healing process.

5. To help ease movement after icing and a hot bath, you can apply one of the many commercial linaments available, such as Ben-Gay.

6. Massage is one of the favorite remedies for sore muscles. It increases the circulation of blood to the sore area and it usually feels great. The East German athletes are given at least one hour of massage therapy per day to speed healing and prevent further injury and to keep their muscles fresh and relaxed. (Rhonda again: Different people have different attitudes toward massage; I love it, while Rich seems to avoid it at all costs. Our culture has not made it exactly easy to accept massage, but we are breaking down some of those barriers and are beginning to understand that massage can offer release from tensions and soreness. It is unfortunate that massage parlors have given the discipline such a bad reputation. Legitimate massage therapists have much to offer the athlete and the average person facing today's stressful world).

7. If you are suffering from muscle soreness, and it is uncomfortable at night to the extent that it keeps you awake, you may want to use a heating pad.

8. Aspirin can also help. (We have differing views on aspirin. Rhonda uses it sparingly, aware that too much aspirin can cause stomach problems. Rich does use it occasionally, especially after a long run, to take down the swelling within his legs and knees. Neither encourage its use too frequently).

9. If your soreness is, in reality, an injury and not merely muscle stiffness, lay off any additional exercise. Take a day off. Even gentle warm-ups may seem like running a marathon to a muscle that is injured. More exercise will only aggravate the problem. You can continue doing exercises that do not involve the use of the affected muscle, but don't push yourself to compounding an injury. You should be able to differentiate between soreness and injury. An ache is usually soreness, while a pain is likely an injury. Caution counts in the exercising game.

IN CONCLUSION

The human machine is cold in the morning. It needs to be

warmed up in order to function properly, just as any other machine does. Being the most sophisticated of machines in the world, the human body should be warmed gently in order to prevent injury. Warming up the human body, however, is not difficult. The warm-up can, and should, lead to additional exercises in order to maintain the human machine in its best possible tune. The warm-up, however, can be used as an end in itself, offering a perfect way to get the body moving first thing in the morning, thereby guaranteeing a body more ready to face the day's activities.

It also guarantees a body much more ready to take the next great steps. Which leads us into the next chapter, where we'll discuss an exercising program that could easily be called "Invisible Exercises," since no one will ever know you're daily becoming fitter and healthier than they are—until you're ready to step into the phone booth, tear open your shirt or blouse, and reveal yourself as Fit-Person.

2

No Fuss Fitness

One rule of physics that seems to have stood up for us over the years because it is so charmingly simple has to do with inertia. The rule is this one: A body at rest tends to remain at rest, until acted upon by some outside force. The phrasing may be a little bit off, but the meaning seems clear.

We've all known people who fit that rule. People who have the ability to, at the least provocation, become "bumps on a log." People who can raise idleness to an art-form. People who, in the face of a world filled with things to do, manage to find a safe little harbor where...nothing happens.

They are the great relaxers, seeming to function on a different set of rules and on a different level of consciousness than the rest of the world. Sometimes they are even amusing, especially in the methods they employ to guarantee their inertia. Virtually every one of them, however, has a hidden capacity for great speed, much like a dozing crocodile that seems almost statue-like—until aroused, threatened or hungry. When motivated by any of those stimuli, the great relaxers are likely to exhibit a speed and dexterity of movement that would startle even The Flash of comic book fame.

The methods of getting them to move are often shrouded in mystery, however.

Many of us go through those periods of languid lethargy during various parts of our lives. It seems that kids suffer a streak of it during summer vacation, only to become highly activated and extremely motivated to have a very good, active, exciting time when the vacation is in its eleventh hour. When asked why they started to enjoy the summer so late, they usually answer with something like, "I was spending June and July and part of August trying to figure out how to do it right." This is from the same kid who, a year before, concluded a four year stint of what appeared to be a very serious combination of hypertension, St. Vitas' dance, and kinetic self-immolation. Even attaching an anchor to him didn't seem to keep him in one place for more than a few minutes.

Everyone seems to oscillate somewhere between the kinetic and the inert, because life is neither on one or the other end of the pendulum. It is a mixed bag, from day to day. We react differently to different days and different motivating factors. We move up and down the scale of activity. Which is why we take such rapt notice of people whose throttles are stuck at one end of the scale or the other, *Maximum Volume* or *Off.*

Most of us regulate our lives by way of motivation. If we are motivated by hunger, we eat. If we are motivated to get to the seashore for the weekend, we plan it out, throw everything into the car, and off we go. If we are motivated to rise within the company where we work, we try a bit harder than the next person and ultimately we reach our goal.

Motivation is a strange critter, though.

Being human, we tend to become motivated more by things that will give us satisfaction pretty quickly. Long-term motivation is not as much fun as short-term motivation because we have to wait around too long for the reward, and man is not the most patient of beasts. There's nothing wrong with that. As long as we don't go through life without long-term goals and are not totally impatient for the quick reward.

To be driving home from work on Friday evening and hear some mention of the seashore on the radio and to become instantly motivated to go to the seashore for the weekend (to the extent that you walk in the door and gather the gang together for an immediate exit to the shore) can be very nice, very spontaneous, and a real adventure—something that you'll probably all talk about for a long time to come, something that you'll probably talk about much longer (and in much more glowing terms) than you would about a weekend at the shore that's been in the planning stages for months.

We tend, though, to need motivations for virtually everything we do. Some of us tend to clean out the junk that accumulated in the back seat of the car only when we know someone is going to be riding there, at which point we find various objects we've been vainly searching for over the past three months.

We tend to put off fitness and health because it demands some direct action on our part.

Health, for as long as anyone can remember, has always been regarded in a negative sense. We've always thought of health as the absence of sickness and disease. In actuality, we should think of health as something we construct and work toward during our lives in conjunction with our bodies, rather than sitting around hoping for it as an alternative to sickness.

Fitness is one way of working toward health.

But we get tired of hearing about that, because we already know it—at least intellectually.

It doesn't take an Einstein to figure out that fitness increases health because it makes the body and mind more able to resist sickness. Big deal, right? A moron can intuit that much.

The problem is to become motivated to want to achieve fitness.

More and more people are working toward fitness these days because they are becoming much more in touch with themselves. They are no longer obsessed only with the work-a-day world. They have moments for leisure, and during those moments, they are taking a good look at themselves and finding that they can do much more with life than their parents could, simply by making sure that the body, the vehicle that carries them through life, is well-tuned and in good working order for the trip. The question becomes one of whether the person wants to go through life driving a school bus, a pick-up truck or a sports car. Some, with great energy stores at their command, manage all three.

Fitness is becoming a very positive thing in our society, and it's a positive thing that cannot help but have good effect upon both individuals and the society these individuals form. End of lecture on that point. Virtually everyone would agree that a fit body is better equipped for the trip through life than a run-down, unhealthy body.

Some very active people, however, seem to have trouble finding time in the day to become fit the way their counterparts do, who manage to find time and motivation for swimming and tennis and racquetball and running and bicycling. Not everyone's interest lies within the lifestyle where showers are taken two and three times a day and where one must consume great amounts of fluid to replace all the sweat used up in the process of staying healthy and fit. Some people who wish to be fit have very active lives in other directions, whether it be going to spectator sports events, puttering around the house on weekends, going to concerts, or using available free time to relax.

For those individuals, it is merely a difference in style, and not so much a difference in motivation. They still want to be fit and by that, healthy, but they don't have the inclination to run five miles at lunch or play three sets of tennis after work or go back-packing every other weekend.

So how do you tone up the muscles and encourage development of important muscle groups? How do you get your wind back after giving it a vacation all these years?

It is all a matter of fitting it in to what you are already doing. It can be done virtually all day long, if you wish, and no one even needs to know you're doing it because you call no attention to yourself.

It is merely a matter of learning how to take advantage of your day as it is now constructed.

What follows are more than a dozen exercises for various parts of your body that you can incorporate into any normal day, exer-cises that can be done indoors, at home or at the office, that will match your motivation toward fitness with your already busy schedule. Exercise that will contribute to your functioning more effectively and efficiently in life, having more energy to enjoy life more thoroughly, and firming up that which may have been falling into the hands of the Inertia Monster.

After you've done your daily fitness fling during the course of your normal day, there's nothing wrong with walking around with a smile on your face—it'll make people wonder what you've been up to, and only you need to know.

FUEL STORED, FUEL USED

Both of us love to eat. I suppose that most Americans do. We are a country of immigrants. Many of our ancestors came to Amer-ica to escape starvation in their own countries. It seems as though, once in America, they made the raising of food a prime priority. America quickly became the world leader—and expert—in produc-ing food. Eating well, and eat often, seems to be an American her-itage which, in itself, is not a sin against nature. We are fighting the urge here to go off on a thousand tangents on food, but we will try to confine ourselves to comments on food as it applies to health and fitness.

Some of our most relaxing moments come over a large pizza with all the fixins and a bottle of wine; we try to relax in that manner at least once a week, often following a workout at the track or an hour-long exercise session in the living room. In order to justify our fixation with pizza and wine at least once a week, we have come up with a basic philosophy: We can eat what we get the urge to eat as long as we keep one step in front of allowing the calories to take up residence. Simply put, keep moving so you burn more calories than you take in.

A desire to lose a few pounds is probably the most cited reason for taking up an exercise program. It may be one of the reasons you purchased this book. You want to drop a few pounds and readjust the remaining pounds into a more favorable arrangement. We should bear one fact in mind when talking about losing pounds: Barring glandular disorder (which is much more rare than people trying to rationalize overweight would like to indicate), weight gain and loss is simply a matter of calories consumed vs. calories used. Because of changes in metabolism within the body, the older you become, the fewer calories you burn just to exist.

The best exercise for weight loss remains the one where you place the palms of your hands against the dinner table and push hard enough to remove yourself from the food. If you want to lose weight, either eat less or move more in order to burn up more of what you do eat. For fitness and weight loss, you'd do better to both eat less and move more. Weight loss by itself does not insure good health or fitness.

Although our bodies derive energy from nutrients in food, eating more food does not necessarily mean more energy—especially for the non-active. On the contrary. Large amounts of energy are used by the body in the digestive processes, especially when dealing with fatty foods. This can leave a person feeling listless and little inclined to move at all. The stomach is pulling so much energy from the body that the alternatives to sitting and letting the stomach do its thing are very limited. You can smile, sigh or belch every once in a while, but even that takes a certain amount of energy.

Consuming smaller, well-balanced meals with lots of roughage (especially as you get older and need more regularity) will leave you with more energy...and you'll be better nourished. Our intention is not to belabor this point, because it is not within the scope of this book to deal heavily with the heavy question of being too heavy; there are shelves of diet books in bookstores, most of them not worth the paper they're printed on, since all diet boils down to is eat less to weigh less, while keeping a balanced diet, and while continuing to do so throughout your life. We will briefly discuss diet and the role food plays in daily life, and then will move on to the exercises for this chapter.

One of the simplest and most effective (but not one of the easiest) exercise one can practice is that of self-control. Consumption of food is as much a result of years of psychological conditioning as it is a physical need. The clock telling us it's mealtime is enough of a learned stimulus to convince most of us that we're hungry, even if food is the farthest thing from our minds at that point. If you were ever in a situation where the clock said it was time to eat, and you were unable to do so, you probably found that the urge to eat vanished once the clock told you that the appointed mealtime was over.

You must learn to differentiate between what you think is hunger and what you know is hunger. Learn to listen to your body so that you can interpret what it is really telling you, as opposed to what you believe it's telling you from a long life of being told that you must eat at certain times of the day or you'll fall victim to dire circumstances. Also, cutting back on food should be done very gradually. A snack here and there vanishing from your daily routine is much more tolerable than going (excuse the pun) cold turkey. You can start the gradual process by eating half portions of your food. When you find yourself going for that extra fried chicken leg, ask yourself: "Do I really need this?" The answer is usually, "No!"

An exercise that may put your eating into its proper perspective is to make a complete list of *everything* you eat each day for two weeks. The list may well reveal some distinct patterns in your eating that should—and could—be broken. The survey of your dietary habits for two weeks could provide valuable insights into why you crave a cookie at 3 p.m.; perhaps a piece of fruit during lunch would have helped you through this programmed hungry period and would have contributed more to good nutrition than a cookie would.

We have a friend who refuses to eat anything after 7 p.m. If he must work late and he doesn't get home in time to eat dinner, he just cancels it out. His next meal, then, is a nutritious breakfast the following day. An extreme solution? Extreme for most people, perhaps, but it works for him. His rule of not eating after 7 p.m. makes sense because since one is usually very inactive in the evening, food eaten after 7 p.m. usually just lays in the stomach and is in no way used by the body because the body is doing nothing to use it. A good rule of thumb (unless you happen to work in the evenings) is that anything eaten after 7 p.m. is guaranteed to turn to fat. Our friend is very trim and does not look as though he's suffered from missing an occasional meal. Most of the unwanted roundness in us comes from evening eating.

As long as our basic nutritional needs are being met, then, we should seriously consider customizing our diets to our real needs. That 3 p.m. cookie might be perfectly fine for a dieting individual who's disciplined enough to know that it's the only sweet they'll treat themselves to all day, so it is needed on schedule to help them psychologically. For someone less disciplined, that one cookie could set the juices flowing to the extent that it could trigger a full-scale eating binge. (Ask Rich about the challenge of eating only one Cheeto.)

What is important for our bodies and our psychological well-being is that we tailor our diet in a fashion sensible enough that we can live with it. Many fad diets exist that promote weight loss, but do not stress sensible eating habits. Dieters overlook the fact that, once the fad diet is through, so is weight loss. Dieting is a full-time proposition. But who would want to go through the rest of his or her life eating only grapefruit and eggs?

The recommended exercises in this chapter will *not* account for a massive amount of weight loss when practiced simply as exercises. Coupled with good nutrition and sensible eating habits, their favorable results will be augmented several times over.

MAKING YOURSELF HABIT-FORMING

If you set one goal here, it should be to lead an active daily life. A moving body gathers less fat. Approach your body—and your life—from a new angle and create new habits: habits that will last you through the years. Breaking old, deeply-rooted habits is not easy. Don't try to do it all in one day; be gentle with yourself. If you were pretty much inactive up to this point, anything you do now is an improvement over the nothing you were doing until today. Patience, again, is a prime word for success.

A woman we know recently told us that she had gone out to run a two and one-half mile Parcourse exercise route at a local community college. "I was out of shape and I knew it," she said, "and I hated every minute of it." No kidding? Our response, we're sorry to say, was not very patient.

If she was out of shape and knew it, what was she doing trying to run two and one-half miles on a Parcourse? No wonder she doesn't like exercise! She doesn't understand what it is, how it works, or what it can do. That tendency to want to improve in a day or screw it is the worst possible attitude to have toward exercise and fitness—and toward life in general.

This word will be repeated over and over and over in this book, regarding the individual exercises and regarding fitness in general: *Patience.* It is a virtue—a virtue that will stand you in good stead for the rest of your life.

In order to further ease you into an exercise program, we've come up with some great exercises for everyday life. Some are mere common sense, some are extremely simple, and most can be done with the greatest of ease. These present adequate opportunity for you to improve the shape you are in without it being a big deal; they also put you on the next plateau before really going overboard and getting into serious exercises on a regular basis. (We use "overboard" in a positive sense here; not falling overboard on an oceanliner, but diving overboard from an overloaded ship that is sinking.) When doing any exercises—or when going through your daily life—good posture and good body mechanics serve to strengthen muscles in your back, arms and legs, and also serve to help prevent injuries to active people.

Incorporating the exercises in this chapter into your daily life will have many benefits. Among the benefits are these:

1. These practices don't require a warm-up period because they are activities that are integrated with your everyday actions.

2. These exercises are not strenuous and therefore need not be reserved for times when you have an empty stomach. They are things that can be done in daily life—and that you may already be doing to a limited extent.

3. They are completely independent of the weather, and do not have to wait for a sunny day.

4. They can be integrated into vacations and weekends and virtually any time you are awake.

5. They serve to establish a good base of exercise and fitness, from which you can mount a charge to the next level of exercising.

6. If you are already engaged in a fairly strenuous exercise routine, these exercises will complement your current exercises, and may also serve to help keep you loose and relaxed so that you can continue your current exercising program minus some of the stiffness.

7. If you are already engaged in a strenuous exercise program, these can easily be substituted into your daily routine on days when your regular rigorous exercise program is impossible. They will tie the muscles over until you can give them another regular workout.

8. Most of them are fun to do—and all are certainly easy to do.

THE NO-FUSS LINE-UP

I. **Walk**—Perhaps the most basic and simple act we perform on a daily basis beyond sleeping. It is undergoing a sort of revival in this country that has fallen (almost logically) on the heels of the running boom. Walking is simple and, done regularly, can be very beneficial to the human body. It can be used rather extensively indoors.

In a building that has elevators, for instance, opting to walk the steps can burn calories and strengthen basic body systems. You wouldn't want to walk the stairs if your office is on the ninety-seventh floor, of course; but if a few flights of steps are involved, you can often beat the elevator to your floor and get some quick exercise in the process. Our building has three stories and an elevator; there are some elderly and handicapped people in the building, so it is very helpful for them, but offers a too-easy temptation for people who are basically healthy and want to stay that way. Luckily, our elevator is one of the world's slowest, so we can easily beat it to our place on the top floor even after coming back from a hard run.

Using the stairs (and this is meant only half-jokingly) makes you familiar with the stairs in your office or apartment or condo building, which is a real plus if the building ever catches fire. Your first inclination will be to go to the stairs. Those who use the elevators will have to pause and ask a question that can be very embarrassing when there's fire and smoke threatening their life: "Where are the stairs?"

Remember, though, that these exercises are not meant to work up a sweat, but merely to encourage your fitness a little at a time. Therefore, unless you are looking for some really strenuous work, walk up the stairs at a casual, comfortable pace, taking slightly deeper breaths than you would while walking on a level surface. Walking stairs is an aerobic activity that is a great way to strengthen your upper legs (quadriceps) and calves. And in addition to burning more calories than walking on the level, it heightens cardiovascular endurance, which serves as a good preparation for later exercises in this book. Stand straight, use the handrails if you need them, and go slowly at first. Pay close attention to your first attempt to walk up a set of stairs; compare the memory of that first day with a day on the same set of steps six weeks later.

Do your daily walking as briskly as possible. Don't drag yourself along, walk with distinction and authority, proving to the world that you know where you're going, even if the rest of the world is a little confused.

Get in the habit of parking your car farther away from where you work or where you shop, thereby forcing yourself to walk a bit farther each day. This will contribute to your fitness in general, and make your other exercising go easier. Remember, what you want to do is to develop new habits. By forcing yourself to walk farther outdoors, you will have yourself in the habit of walking indoors, instead of asking someone else to do your walking for you, or instead of just not getting up at all when you need or want something from some other place in your home.

By doing more walking where it's practical, you can be two giant steps ahead on the road to fitness and health.

II. Stomach Control—No, this is not a rehashing of what we've already discussed on holding yourself back from your urges to eat food when you don't need it. This has to do directly with your stomach muscles.

While waiting on customers, sitting at your desk or sewing machine, standing at the Xerox machine or filing cabinets, preparing meals, ironing, sitting in your car at a red light, or doing just about anything, you can strengthen your stomach muscles. All you need do is casually tense the muscles of your stomach, tightening them; do it over and over and over during the day, at any possible opportunity. The object is to make it a habit so that you do it frequently during the day. Unless you are modeling two-piece bathing suits in a department store window, no one will ever know you're doing it. Perhaps as a start, you could do it every half-hour, or every time you hear a certain commercial on the radio, or every time you get the urge to look for something to eat.

By tensing the stomach muscles, you are toning, tightening and shortening them. It is an excellent way to improve posture and to better carry any extra weight that you may have. We've all seen men who look as though they are pregnant or as though they ate hand grenades that exploded in their stomachs. That condition doesn't have to exist. It is a combination of spreading fat and weak stomach muscles. Tighten 'em up now.

This is perhaps the best place to interject the simple fact that good nutrition can go a long way in making stomach muscle development easier and in giving you a flatter-looking stomach. Good nutrition includes plenty of roughage, those foods that keep things (i.e., food) moving through your system. It keeps your intestines free of excess waste products, thereby promoting a flat stomach and eliminating (no pun) those feelings of lethargy associated with your digestive tract working overtime. Additionally, keeping yourself regular by using roughage helps cut down on the incidence of cancer in the lower tract, the theory being that matter residing too long in the intestines are perfect breeding grounds for bacteria.

III. Tucked in Buttocks—Very similar to holding in your stomach, tucking in the buttocks is one of those things you rarely do, but could incorporate into your day with great ease. Essentially, all it involves is putting a little firmness into them by tightening them whenever possible so that there is some muscle development there, instead of allowing them to become soft and consequently to droop. This is most easily done in the standing position and goes unnoticed, unless you're in a bathing suit at the time. If you want to remain subtle about it, you won't want to do it while walking.

The tightening of the buttocks is terrific both for the buttocks and for the hamstrings. You can combine this one with the previous exercise for the stomach and thereby accomplish twice as much in half the time.

IV. Squat—Did you drop something on the floor? Need something from a shelf near the floor? Putting something away at knee-level? Don't bend at the waist to reach it. First of all, to do so is bad body mechanics. You increase the chance of injury when you bend at the back. But more importantly, squatting is great exercise for your upper thighs. Keep your back straight when squatting and don't use the back to do the work. Use those thighs; feel the stretching when you push yourself back to a standing position!

V. Calf Stretch—Don't attempt to do this one with high heels and platform shoes. In fact, wearing high heels and platform shoes is not a really good idea in the first place, but we won't get into that here.

This one is a very easy exercise that can be done discreetly and gently. Standing with your feet together, raise and lower yourself on your toes. It's a very good way to stretch and strengthen your lower leg muscles. Do this one ten times, or as many times during the day as you feel inclined. It can also be incorporated into reaching toward high shelves; it gives the calves good definition and added strength and flexibility.

VI. Stretch—Stretch, don't strain. There's a very marked difference.

Need something on the top shelf? Or across that counter? Try stretching for it yourself before you call someone else to do it. You can feel the satisfying stretch in your back and arms. Incorporate stretching those calves into this one. Even if you know you're not going to be able to reach what you want, you should at least try.

Incidentially, restrooms provide us with the privacy we're not always afforded in public places. If you feel you might draw attention to yourself by doing any one of these or one of your own inventions, escape to a stall or incorporate it with your visit to the restroom by doing a few deep-knee bends before you exit the stalls. It takes some practice, but you'd be surprised where you can fit in a little exercise.

VII. Head Roll—A simple and effective exercise tool that can be a great tension reducer is the head roll. Take a short break from what you are doing, sit up straight in your chair, close your eyes and relax. Concentrate on becoming loose. Take several slow, deep breaths and let your head slowly fall forward. Feel that pressure in the back of your neck? Now, slowly, gently, rotate your head to the left, toward the back, to the right, and then return it to the front. Do this at least twice. Now repeat, going in the opposite direction. Do this as often as you need or want to have the relaxing effect during the day. It feels good, and can also help head off tension headaches if you get into the habit of doing it at the first hint of tension.

VIII. Squeezing of the Balls—A handy little thing to keep laying around the house or in your desk drawer or your locker is a squeeze ball of some sort. A golf ball would suffice, or you can check out what's available in a toy store. A tennis ball is too large.

Play with the ball during the day by squeezing it while you're reading the paper at home or reviewing some material at the office. It's a great strengthening exercise for the forearms and also helps relieve tension.

Why do you want to strengthen the forearms? To help you

Squat

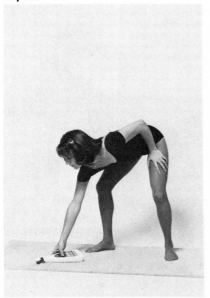

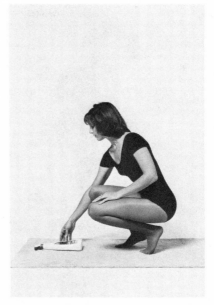

This is the wrong way to pick something up from the floor; bad for the back.

Use up a few more calories by squatting to pick something up from the floor.

Calf Stretch

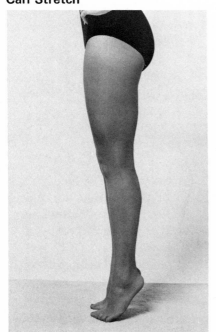

The calf stretch can be effected any time you raise yourself on your toes, whether it's reaching for something beyond your reach on a shelf or doing it strictly as an exercise. Listen to your muscles when you do this one. Don't stretch too far and don't bounce. Make it smooth and simple and don't hold it too long—no sense pushing it to the verge of a cramp. Balancing on high heels does not have the same effect; instead of making the muscle supple, high heels shorten it and make it tight.

Head Roll

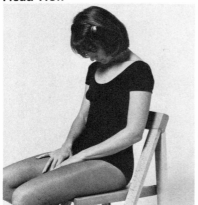

Sit down relaxed, and let your head fall forward onto your chest.

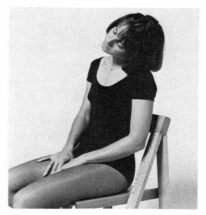

Now, roll your head, very relaxed, toward the left.

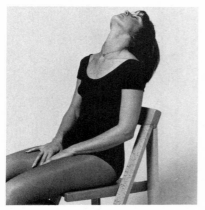

Continuing the rolling motion, bring the head back, relaxed and flaccid.

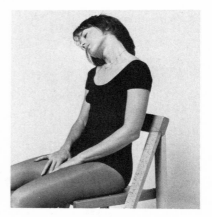

Continue the rolling motion to the right, returning the head to the chest.

carry all those parcels and grocery bags by yourself, of course. Try not to rely on your husband or wife or the children to help you carry things. Be very positive about this. Really. Unloading all those things from the car and carrying them back and forth to and/or from the house is work. And you hate it, right? Of course you do. And you know why? You're tired or you're slightly out of shape. We don't urge you to court exhaustion overexerting yourself, though. And we *don't* want you to do so much at one time that you get turned off toward getting back in shape. So again, begin slowly. If you've only been accustomed to carrying two grocery bags at a time, try three. Just don't crush the potato chips.

Don't take your car if your destination is within walking distance. The combined effect of walking and carrying parcels is great exercise. (Just don't do too much at one time. If you are a woman weighing one hundred five pounds, don't carry a twenty pound frozen turkey in one arm and a sixty pound bag of potting soil in the other arm and then walk a mile to your house. Use your common sense. You should do just enough so that you feel a bit of an effort in the arms.)

Remember, you're not attacking all this at once. You're gradually changing your habits for life. The effects of all these small changes are cumulative and will dove-tail nicely with each other. The result will eventually be increased strength and energy levels that will be with you throughout the day.

IX. Standing on Your Own Two Feet—A minor tidbit: Standing burns more calories than sitting. If you find yourself in situations where it is as convenient to stand as to sit, stand. It will also offer you more of an opportunity to use some of the practices we've already mentioned, especially the calf stretch.

X. Knee Lifts—While sitting at your desk studying, or at the kitchen table writing out checks to pay the bills, or at the office typing, give your back, abdomen and upper legs some strengthening by bringing yourself almost out to the edge of your chair. Place your feet flat on the floor. Tilt back some while you straighten your back and raise your legs at the knees. Hold them there for as long as you can. Once you've practiced this one a few times, you'll be able to do it without even interrupting the work you're doing. Think what an accomplishment it will be to exercise while continuing to type or sew.

XI. For Women Only—You can improve the muscle tone in your bustline while sitting around passing the time. It's easy and a sure chest-tightener. Grasp your right wrist with your left hand in front of your chest, and your left wrist with your right hand. Now, try to pull them apart to the count of ten. Next, join palm to palm in front of you, fingers to the ceiling in the classic praying pose; now push the palms against each other to the count of ten. Alternate the two, pull and push, while watching television or at any time you have a free sixty seconds. (Actually, we were only joking with the "For Women Only" title of this one; the same exercise is very good for men who want to tone their chests.)

Knee Lift

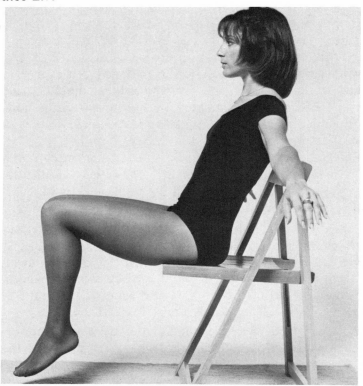

Do this one especially smoothly, holding the legs together and raising them in unison; hold as long as you can.

For Women Only

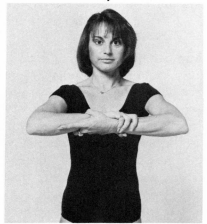

Grasp your wrists and pull against them trying to pull them apart.

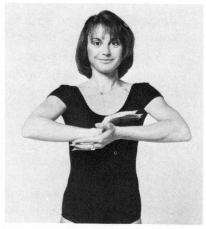

Place heel of palm against heel and push, as pictured, or in prayer pose.

XII. The Watchers and the Listeners—Some exercises lend themselves to being done while you are watching television or listening to the stereo. They don't require a great deal of attention, so you can do them and watch your favorite program at the same time, thereby accomplishing two things simultaneously, something that is only too rare in life. By being the master of your own exercise program, you won't have to wait until the regularly scheduled television exercise shows; your exercise is at your command, rather than you being a slave to a programming time slot.

From the stereo front, we've both found that some exercises are much more easily done to music, which either helps you keep time or just entertains you while you stretch in the privacy of your own home.

XIII. The Butterfly—Sit on the floor. With your back straight, join the soles of your feet. Hold feet together by grasping them with both hands. Now flutter your knees quickly, 1-2-3. Begin again and repeat this series ten times. Following this, grasp your ankles and press your elbows down upon your thighs firmly. Don't push it beyond gentle stretching; if it begins to hurt, back off. When you are finished fluttering, maintain position and see how close you can bring your nose to your toes. You'll probably be tight at first. This one takes quite a bit of practice and patience, but is excellent for the groin and hips.

Butterfly

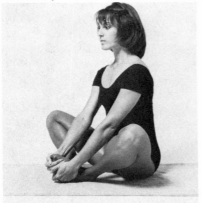
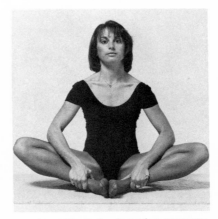

Keep your back straight and your soles together; now flutter your knees up and down.

At the end of the fluttering sequence, grasp ankles and press down on thighs with elbows.

Leg Stretch—With your back straight, still sitting on the floor from the previous exercise, keep the left leg drawn to your groin and hold it with the left hand. Keep the right leg flexed and grasp the sole of the right foot with the right hand. Raise and straighten the right leg out from the body a total of five times. Switch and do the same on the other side.

Leg Stretch II—Bend the left leg so your foot is next to your left buttock and extend the right leg in front of you. Gently grasp the right ankle with both hands. Bend forward to touch your nose to your right knee in a gentle bouncing fashion; repeat ten times. Now, do the same with the other leg.

Now, join your two legs together in front of you, grasp the ankles gently and attempt to touch your nose to the knees. Notice, we used the word *attempt*. Chances are that you won't make it all the way. That's just fine. With patience, you will manage it or you'll at least begin coming closer with each try. Do not hurt yourself trying too hard to do it now. This one offers great benefits to the calves, Achilles tendon and the hamstrings.

Leg Stretch

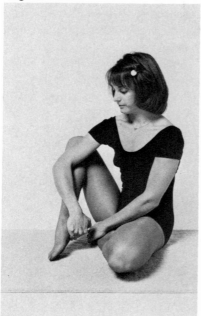 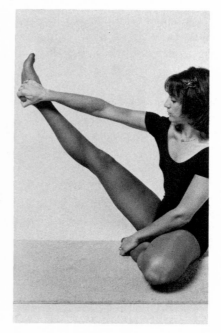

The secret of this one is to remain re-laxed, and therefore loose.

Pick up the leg only as high as it will com-fortably go. Don't strain.

Leg Stretch II

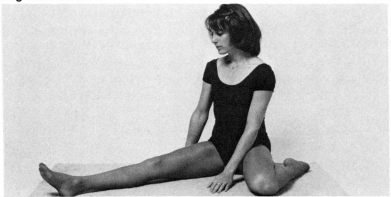

Don't strain when you begin this one, but try to keep leg straight.

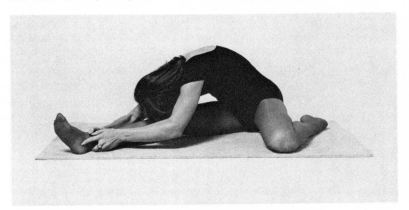

Don't despair if you can't touch head to knee on first try.

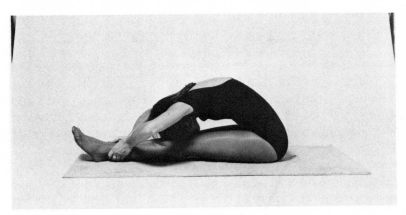

Keep the legs straight, and bow at the waist, staying relaxed.

XIV. Leg Raise—While lying flat on your back, with your arms out to your sides, draw your knees up to your chest; next, straighten them above you to the count of five; then, lower them (together) slowly to the floor. Repeat this five times. As you get stronger, gradually add one more repetition until you reach ten. When you've mastered that, drop back to five and don't rest the legs on the floor between repetitions. This is good for the hamstrings and great for your stomach, especially when you don't touch the floor with your legs.

XV. Hip Roll—Lie on your back and draw your knees up to your chest. Keep your arms straight out to your sides, with palms down flat on the floor. Now, roll to the left, return to the center, then roll to the right. This whole process counts as one. Repeat ten times. You'll feel it in your stomach and your upper arms as they stabilize you while you turn. This one is a little more obvious than some of the more subtle ones, but your kids will think you're playing with them and will enjoy it, and if you're on the floor watching television, it's a great one to do while the commercials are on; you can be getting fit while they're trying to sell you food stuffs you don't need.

XVI. Shower Stretch—Did you ever notice that, unless you are showering with someone who can help you, there are certain areas of your back that never get scrubbed because they seem impossible to reach? That need no longer be the case. Your back can now be as clean as the rest of you and you'll increase your shoulder flexibility in the process.

Hold the face cloth in your left hand and raise it over your left shoulder with the palm of your hand facing your back. Now bring your right hand to meet your left hand (or at least to grasp the end of the face cloth) by bending it back from below at the waist with the palm of the hand facing out. Now scrub the upper left quadrant of your back with primarily your left hand, in a sawing motion. Pass the cloth (some people prefer a loofa mit) to the right hand, which has been getting a good workout while waiting, and scrub the lower left quadrant. Keep your left hand where it is while you do this. Relax. Now do the other side by reversing the process. Your back will never lack for attention again.

Upon completion of the process, let the cloth drop into the tub or shower floor, and join your hands behind your back, stretching the arms back gently. Repeat the process from the other side, reversing hands. (Learning how to do this guarantees you'll never

Leg Raise

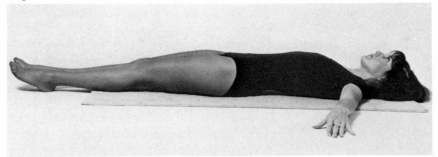

This one is extremely easy; enjoy the sensation of lying flat.

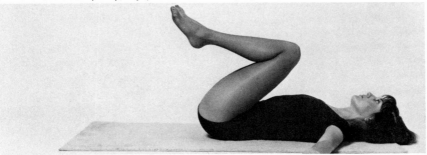

Try to keep your upper body flat throughout the entire exercise.

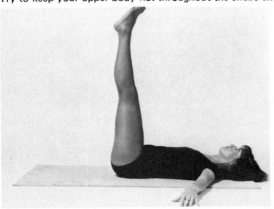

Raise the legs straight toward the ceiling, upper body still.

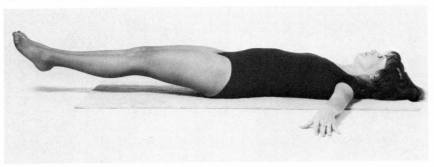

Now the difficult part; hold the heels a few inches above the floor.

Hip Roll

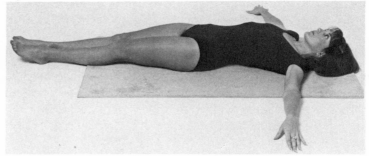

Again, begin this one by lying perfectly flat on the floor.

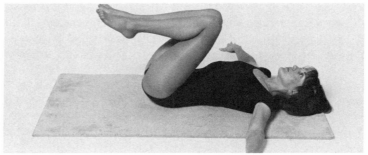

Now, just like the previous exercise, raise the knees toward chest.

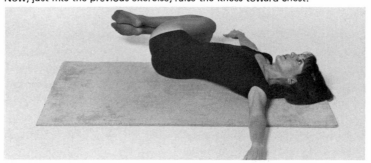

Keeping the knees together, roll them toward your right, smoothly.

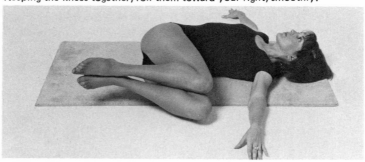

Now, roll them toward the left, doing all the rolling off the hips.

have an itch you can't scratch. Now talk about independence!)

XVII. More Life in Sex—Some people contend that they can't exercise because they are coming off a long, hard night. By incorporating some exercise into your long, hard nights, they needn't be anything but more enjoyable. One activity that can take up some time at night and that can be further enhanced by exercise, is intimacy between partners. Remember that fitness enhances your energy stores, and those stores can be called upon at the darndest times.

Exercising can be fit into almost any activity, and none better than love-making. Working up a healthy sweat while exercising with someone special can be a very sensuous experience, and can lead to other physical activities. Showering together in that steaming water followed by a mutual gentle or vigorous massage can be the perfect prelude to further intimacy.

One common non-Victorian practice in contemporary love-making is for the female to assume a mounted position with her partner on his back. This affords her an excellent opportunity to give her thighs and buttocks a serious workout. Conventionally, females tend to rest back on the thighs of their partners and/or

Shower Stretch

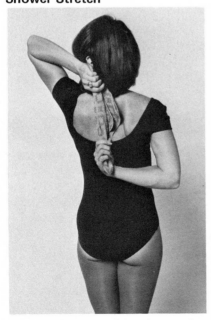 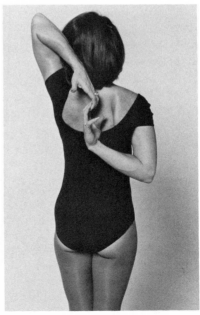

Use a wash cloth until you become flexible enough to join hands.

Make sure to try this under a warm shower, to keep yourself loose.

More Life in Sex

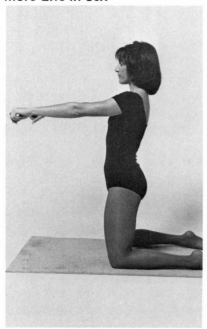

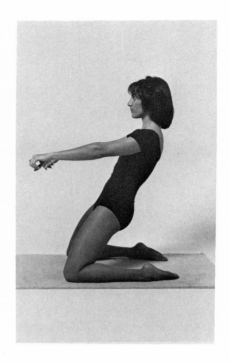

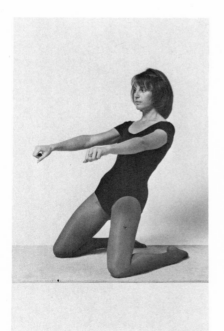

This is a terrific exercise for the thighs. It puts very good stress on the foreparts of the legs, firming and toning them. It can be used very easily as a straight exercise, or can be incorporated into your sex techniques. Besides freeing the hands for other things, it offers an exercise in control and dexterity. This is one exercise where even when practice makes perfect, it is still fun to keep practicing.

lean forward, supporting themselves on their partners' shoulders, or a combination of both. Why not try that position while using neither of those crutches? Using your partner's thighs as little as possible for support, use a "Look, Ma, no hands" technique, giving your thighs a good workout. At the same time, you can tighten the gluteal and abdominal muscles, which will offer additional help in firming up the buttocks and stomach, while also heightening sensations during love-making.

By experimenting with holding other positions, a great deal of enjoyment can be derived from your love-making that was not evident before. Being fit should also allow you to more fully enjoy love-making and to enjoy it more often.

IN CONCLUSION

Without overstating the message of this chapter, we'd like to leave it very simply: Think fitness in your daily life. The orientation to fitness will be as good for your psyche and self-esteem as it will be for your body. Use your imagination to come up with exercises precisely fit for your home, office and sex-life. This is merely a starting point. Flow with the exercises, and pretty soom your daily life will seem just a bit empty if you forget them.

The next section features a more standardized routine, but using household items that can be adapted very easily. They are also exercises that can be a great deal of fun to do. Instead of being in the bag, fitness is in the bucket.

3

The Bucket Brigade

We have a good friend who is a boon to future archaeologists and to modern sporting goods salesmen.

Long after our civilization is dead and gone, archaeologists will begin poking through the rubble, looking for clues to what made us tick during our tenure. They'll find libraries housing all the knowledge of the world, they'll find McDonalds and will learn how we streamlined our methods of eating after many years of experimenting, and they'll find our friend's den, where they'll learn more than they want to know about the subject of participant sports.

To open the door to his den is to take your life in your own hands. It ranks with climbing the north face of the Matterhorn, parachuting from a Skyhook-type balloon stalled at 104,500 feet, and eating a thick and juicy hamburger while treading water in a shark tank. To open the door of the den is to precipitate an avalanche of every piece of hardware and software ever conceived for the sporting world. He claims that there is a sofa in the room, but no one has ever seen it because all characteristics of the room are hidden by pile upon pile of sporting goods.

He has made many a salesman ecstatic on his periodic sprees. So much so that he gets Christmas cards from sporting goods salesmen from as far away as Hawaii and Alaska. He has more calendars than a bank, because every second or third sporting goods shop in America remembers him—and if he keeps going, he'll have gotten to all the other shops that he's missed to date.

His den is filled with softball bats, first-baseman mitts, volleyballs, tennis balls, soccer shoes, bicycling jerseys, bicycles (one-speed, three-speed, ten-speed and twelve-speed), running shoes (at least fifteen pair), wooden golf clubs (you can see how long his obsession has been on the make), some bent pieces of a hang-glider, etc., etc., etc.

Obviously, he is a doer. Unfortunately, he is not a stick-wither.

He takes a shine to virtually every sport that he sees or hears about, becomes excessively enthusiastic, and runs around like a crazyman buying equipment, practicing, reading up on the rules and the techniques, learning all the names of those who are proficient in the sport (in case he should ever walk into a restaurant or a men's room and find one of them there, he wants to be able to recognize him, get his autograph and shoot the bull with him about his family, batting average, etc.), making his own scoring charts and league standings charts in a loose-leaf notebook. (Oh, yes, he was a vice-grip on at least seventy-eight percent of the world's market of navy blue three-ring binders, all of which he keeps in his attic, each dedicated to a division in a different sport.)

We once made the mistake of asking him which sport was his favorite. He raised his hand to his chin, scratched his head with his free hand, and has still not answered us. I suspect that when the answer comes, it will be something extremely profound, such as, "Well, the sport that I'm playing at the time, I suppose."

Right.

We've always felt that physical-activities-for-fun (as opposed to physical-activities-to-earn-a-living) should be fun, and to us, fun should be spelled u-n-c-o-m-p-l-i-c-a-t-e-d. And i-n-e-x-p-e-n-s-i-v-e.

If you've got to load the car up with two and one-fourth tons of equipment, by the time you get to where you're going to have fun, the fun is all drained out of you in the form of work-type sweat and exertion. You'll be too tired to have fun.

This is not to say that all sports that require a lot of equipment are junk. What it says is, why complicate something more than it has to be? As kids, the best ball games we ever had were the impromptu games where a bunch of scruffy kids in equally scruffy clothes would have one bat, one very much tired and taped hardball, and perhaps three gloves (one for the pitcher, one for the catcher, and one for the first-baseman) between a dozen of us. Once it got organized and we had uniforms and coaches and rules that you couldn't make up as you went along, it lost some of its charm and fun.

There is that, and there is the fact that many sports don't allow you to use up any great amount of calories or to get/stay in shape. In baseball, you can play right field and the nearest you get to exercise is walking out to your position at the beginning of the inning and walking back to the dugout after three outs. You can conceivably spend the whole game without getting within fifty yards of the ball. Let's face it, it's the pitcher's job to see that the ball doesn't get near you. What kind of fun or exercise is that? You could have accomplished as much by not being there at all. You could have gone down to your workshop, taken a piece of plywood, cut it out in a silhouette of yourself, wrapped your uniform around it, and stood it in right field, for all the good you did there. Baseball isn't very good exercise, unless you happen to be a pitcher's arm, a catcher's arm, a catcher's legs, an ump's right or left arm, or a third-base coach's mouth. That's why baseball players spend so much time in spring training lying on the ground doing exercises, because that's all of the exercise they're going to get all season and they have to make at least a pose of being in shape. People who play sports are supposed to be in shape, you know? A few calesthentics at Ft. Lauderdale before the baseball season starts go a long way; the publicity man for the ball club invites all the sports photographers out to take pictures of the ball-players touching their toes—or trying to, and that's all you see in the newspapers in the spring. A bunch of uniformed guys on a big lawn touching their toes.

(Fortunately, the times are changing in some ways. The Los Angeles Dodgers are heavy into running to get in shape, and some of the guys are actually getting pretty darn good at it. They claim that it shows up to their advantage in double-headers, where they are still going strong in the second game while the other guys are beginning to look as though they lost a quarter on the field.)

A person who wants to become proficient at exercising, and by that, become toned and fit, does not have to commit him or herself to roping off one room of the house or apartment to hold all the apparatus that's needed. If you've got a broom closet, you already have space for what you'll need. And, better still, everything you are going to use for this set of exercises can be found or used around the house, either before or after you use it to exercise.

All you need is the following:

- one plastic wash bucket, with handle (in whatever color turns you on)
- one eight-foot piece of laundry line
- two sixty-four ounce plastic bottles (with handles) of liquid laundry detergent

- one bath towel (that has seen better days)
- one tape measure (which can be borrowed or stolen from a sewing kit)
- one spiral binder notebook (a steno or newspaper reporter type is best)
- one pen
- one copy of this book
- one bicycle innertube (used)
- one standard broom

Everything following the bucket (except the broom) can be kept in the bucket, and the bucket can be kept in the broom closet. (Don't put it in the den, as things in the den tend to draw other things to them like great magnets. You don't want a den that's going to attract archaeologists.)

ASSESSING THE MACHINE

Before we get heavily into our bucket brigade exercises, which are more vigorous than the daily routine already covered, some mention should be made regarding the physical shape we're in as we approach this new regime.

As we know, Abe Lincoln notwithstanding, not everyone is created equal—at least not physically. Each of us has varied and different physical capabilities. Some of you may have a medical file two feet long that contains details of some disease or the other, perhaps heart disease or a lung condition. There may also be abnormalities of the spine. On the other hand, you may be one of the fortunate people who has never seen the inside of a doctor's office. Or, you may be the average person, who has gone through life to this point with what we refer to as the normal childhood diseases. Things like mumps or chicken pox and such.

Each of us, however, ages every day, and, in its way, aging is a disease. Therefore, each of us suffers from at least one disease—an incurable one. Aging wears down certain body systems, so even if you have never been to a doctor in your life, there are still systems within your body that are wearing down that may indicate that some caution should be taken in embarking on an exercise program.

It is our feeling that anyone over the age of thirty should have regular annual checkups—extensive checkups. Especially if you are going to be beginning a strenuous exercise program, it would be good to assess where your body stands so that you will better be able to judge exactly how fast and how far you should push it. Harking back to the body as a machine, you would certainly make a thorough examination of your car before taking a long trip, right? You might even go so far as to drop it by your local service station to have a complete checkup before a vacation trip. You owe your body the same consideration.

We urge you to see your physician before getting into strenuous exercise, then. The physician you see should be committed to good physical health habits. Have him give you a thorough checkup. Tell him or her what your goals are. Ask for recommendations based on factors such as your age, weight, and any health-related problems you might have had. You'll have more peace of mind knowing what things you should or shouldn't be attempting. The object of the exercise program is to improve your well-being and not to head you for an early grave. Just as you wouldn't take a beautifully restored Packard on a race down the Baja Peninsula, we don't want to encourage you to get yourself into trouble.

Unfortunately, we've seen some doctors who are overweight, smoke cigarettes and look like the last phase of death, advising perfectly sound people that they shouldn't exercise—it's bad for them. Seek out a sports and fitness oriented physician and get a checkup. You'll go through the rest of this book, and the rest of your life, with a relaxed approach—because you'll know that you are capable of reaching your goals without injury to your body.

BUCKET POWER

I. Notebook, Pen and Tape Measure—People have kept records of virtually everything since the invention of language. Before language, there was picture writing. If you lived in a cave and had killed two bears, you came back, and while you gnawed on the bear meat, you made drawings of two bears on the cave wall; you might embellish it with a sun if it was a sunny day when you killed the bears, and you might also put yourself into the picture. On a day five months hence, when your hunt came up empty, or when the bear just about took your arm off, you could go back to the cave and recall, through the drawings, the day you put away two bears single-handedly.

It is an excellent idea to embark upon the hunt for better fitness and health armed with a record of your progress. Your progress can—and should—be recorded every day. It does not have to be anything fancy or involved. On a daily basis it might only contain a record of how many of a certain exercise you did with a one-line notation on how you felt and how the exercises progressed. Once a week you might include such things as weight (which should be taken first thing in the morning, no clothes, and on an empty stomach), your goals (and be realistic; if you're a size twelve now, you will not fit into that size nine dress for that wedding in two weeks; constantly update and reassess your goals in your notebook), and the measurements of selected areas of the body. You should take measurements of prime parts of the body when you start your program. These areas include:

- underarm (See photograph)
- chest (Measured with the back straight)
- waist
- stomach (See photograph)
- hips
- thighs (To be measured while standing straight with legs spread slightly)
- calves (Again, to be measured with legs spread slightly)
- ankles
- upper arms (Both right and left; measured with arms straight out to sides)
- weight and height should also be measured

Everyone will measure themselves a little bit differently. Don't let that worry you, so long as you measure yourself in a consistent way each time you take the measurements.

You should also consider using your notebook as a personal daily journal of sorts—a kind of diary. Include in it feelings and thoughts about anything that seems important to you at the time, especially those pretaining to your physical well-being. It can be "had a terrific workout today; felt renewed after a tough day." Or it might read "terrible workout; felt sluggish and sore; need a hot bath." By doing this, you'll be able to more accurately appreciate your hard work once you've gotten six months under your belt and you're farther down the road to fitness than ever before in your life; you can go back and read the early entries and you can become reinspired to continue on your path to improvement.

We have constructed a typical notebook for you in the appendix section.

II. A Copy of This Book—An excellent place to actually begin your strenuous program is to assess what about your physical being

Taking Measurements

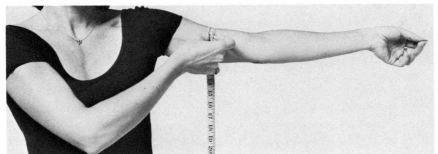

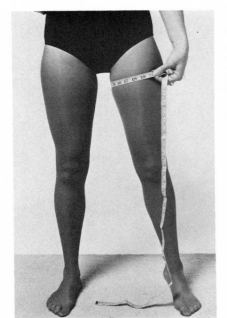

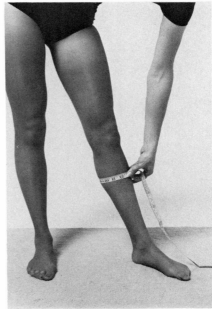

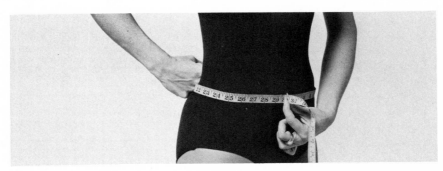

Cont. Next Page

Taking Measurements (cont'd)

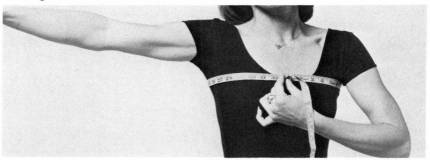

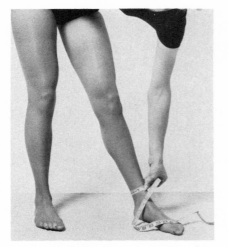

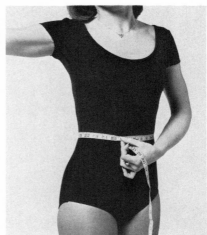

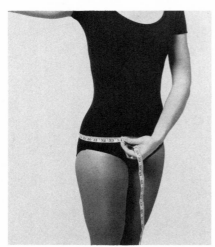

The important thing to keep in mind when taking measurements is to establish a method that can be easily duplicated each time that you do measure yourself, so that you get an accurate reflection of how much you have lost or shifted between each measurement period.

could benefit from a few less pounds and inches. Which areas concern you the most? Start on areas you'd most like to see changed, and in the process, some of the marginal areas will begin to come along on their own.

Stand nude in front of your mirror. If it's a full-lingth mirror, so much the better. Study your curves and bulges carefully. Consider where you would like to have them, or where you would like to remove them. Turn sideways, examining each side view in its turn. Don't cheat and pull your stomach in. Stand as you normally would.

A good mirror is supposed to be sending back an eighty-five percent reflection. Unless you have a trick circus mirror, what you see is what you have to work with. There are certain aspects that you cannot change. Things like height and bone structure. What your job is, then, is to customize and modify what you can change—and what you want to change. Don't be too hard on yourself. That's the body that's gotten you this far in life, and that can take you lots farther. If you were perfect, there'd be no challenge—and that would be pretty dull and boring. And besides, nature, gravity and time has a way of catching up to even those bodies we think are perfect. Turn sideways again as you view yourself. Now, carefully stand with your head up, back straight, shoulders back, and pull that stomach in. Not nearly as bad, huh? And all those changes were accomplished by merely changing your posture.

No one's body is perfect. Even public figures who are noted for their physical attributes often possess little physical idiosyncracies that they've spent their lives trying to change—but without success. Your goal should be to become not someone you aren't, but the best possible person that you can be with what you have to work with. We are trying to change the single major deterent to physical well-being: Inertia. In the process, we can't help but tighten up and lose a few pounds over a period of time (as long as we don't go on an accompanying eating binge).

Now that you've had that long, serious look in the mirror, set some realistic goals in your mind—and in your notebook.

Again assume the pose you took while standing at attention in the mirror. Place your copy of this book (or perhaps a larger and heavier book) on your head. This is an age-old method of improving posture that really works. With the book in place, maintain your posture and walk across the room and back. Can you do it with no problem? Or are you grumbling that flat-heads have an advantage on this one? Try walking around the house with the book perched on your head. It very quickly makes you conscious of your body posture. See if you can keep it balanced there while you read the paper or watch television or have lunch. Besides making you very much aware of your everyday movements, it should also serve to help smooth some of the rough edges from your movements around the house. See how the book on your head fits with your wardrobe; you may want to keep it there indefinitely and be part of a new trend in fashion.

III. Jump Rope—Jumping rope is something that is very much associated with childhood. The rich kids had jump ropes with fancy handles made of colored wood. The rest of us cut up our mothers' old clothesline and tied knots in the ends so that when our palms got slippery, the rope would not go flying. Well, jump rope isn't only for kids. Dr. Ken Cooper, whose book *Aerobics* started a wave of exercisers spreading across the land at the end of the 1960s, rates continuous rope jumping right in there with swimming and running and bicycling as an exercise that builds the all-important cardiovascular system of the body. For those of us who are a little uncoordinated, of course, jump rope can be as much of a challenge at this point in life as it was when we were children; the primary difference is that our bones are more brittle and likely to break now that we are older.

Some people are naturally adept at rope jumping, though. Some of them can do tricks with the rope, never missing a beat, turning it into an art form. Some boxers can skip rope better than they can fight. Jump rope is an exercise that develops the heart and lungs, that strengthens both the thighs and the calves, and that developes the arms and chest and the coordination.

Besides trying to coordinate when to jump with when to swing the rope, the most difficult part of jumping rope for an adult will be in finding a safe place in which to do it. If you have a garage and it isn't all filled with junk, you've got a perfect place. If you aren't shy, you can venture outside to the front porch. But this book deals with the indoors. And where can you safely swing a rope and jump over it without bringing down all the good china? Good question.

If, like us, you live in an apartment, there is no good place to do it. The nearest we can come to a good spot is the balcony. Being on the third floor in an apartment building and jumping rope can cause strained relations with the people who live under you. There is, however, a solution. And that is to purchase one of those smooth plastic sheets that you push under a desk at the office so that the casters on the chair don't get caught up in the shag rug. They can often be purchased second-hand at a used office furniture store and they provide an excellent surface upon which to let the rope glide on each pass, as well as providing protection to your floor. To cut down on the noise of the jumping, place sponges under the plastic at regular intervals; you can purchase a whole bag of plastic sponges at a variety store for as little as $1.29.

Jumping rope should be done carefully at first. As you get more used it it, you'll find you're able to do it in a relatively small space in your home. You'll have complete control of where the rope goes when you swing it, and your lights and book shelves will be completely safe.

Do not try to do too much at one time when you jump rope. Let your breathing be your guide. Don't push yourself to the point that you are gasping or in distress. Remain relaxed and in control. Don't get fancy unless, like riding a bicycle, it begins coming back to you from your childhood.

In your journal, you'll want to note how easy or difficult you found jump rope after all these years. Enter how long (in seconds or minutes) you were able to comfortably continue. These records will be very real proof of your improvement. We tend to minimize our accomplishments and if left unrecorded, we'll be left unable to fully appreciate those extra fifteen seconds we lasted today. And they *do* matter, because they accumulate over the years.

Once you feel comfortable with the jump rope, it is not something that need only be done in the privacy of your home. (Rhonda here: One of the vivid memories from my childhood was both my parents coming out to jump rope with all the neighborhood kids that were jumping their little brains out in the middle of our dead-end street. Use it as an opportunity to get to be with your kids, or nieces or nephews, or the neighborhood kids. And don't feel silly about doing it as an adult. Some simple pleasures never lose their appeal).

IV. Bucket Exercises—Reload all your goodies from this chapter (except the broom) into your bucket.

Now, find a table or a bureau that is strong enough to hold your weight, place the towel on top, and then sit on the towel. Suspend the bucket from your left ankle as your legs hang over the edge. (You might want to wear a pair of socks so the bucket handle doesn't irritate or pinch your skin.) With your back straight, stomach in, stabilize yourself by placing your hands on the table.

Now, raise the bucket to a point where your leg is out straight. Repeat this ten times. This strengthens the quadriceps. Transfer the bucket to the other foot and repeat the exercise.

To strengthen your hamstrings, perform the same exercise while lying on the table or bureau on your abdomen. Don't let the knees hang off the end of the table, though. If you can, balance the bucket handle on the bare sole of your foot and flex your leg. This version is difficult and takes some coordination in placing the bucket handle on your foot. If the bucket is too heavy, merely remove some of the objects until it is a weight that you can work with.

You can also use the bucket filled with the various objects to build up the tone in your arms by sitting on a chair and, resting your elbow on your knee, grasping the bucket handle in your hand and curling your forearm up toward your chest.

The towel can be used, of course, to dry your hands and to wipe away any perspiration. It should not, however, be used in the traditional athletic sense: Don't throw in the towel; keep at it.

Bucket Exercise

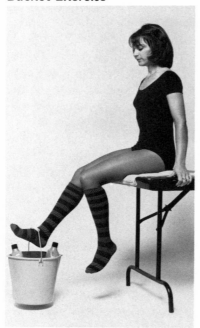

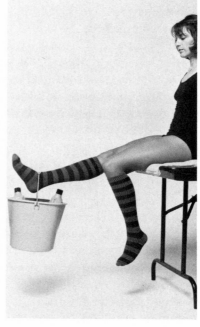

Make sure that the counter or table you use is capable of holding your weight.

Use socks so that the handle does not irritate your ankle.

V. The Broom Stick—If a new broom sweeps clean, you'll really be cleaning up in the inches with this one. The broom can be used to tighten up the waistline and firm the stomach.

Stand with your feet about twelve to eighteen inches apart. Place the broom across your shoulders and rest your arms over it, as though you had been porting two buckets of water up from the wells in Holland. (See the photographs.) With your stomach held in, look straight ahead. Rotate left at the waist, bringing the left arm back and the right arm forward. Keep looking forward. The broom will keep your arms straight. Now return to center and continue on to the right side without pausing. These motions should all be executed smoothly as one. Continue until you've done ten of them. Stop and take two or three deep breaths.

Maintain the same position. Now bend at the waist toward the left and come back up and bend to the right. Try to get down far enough so that you can touch your knee with the broom. Repeat this one ten times and as you progress, increase both exercises to fifteen and then to twenty repeats.

Now, bend at the waist, keeping the legs straight. The broom should still be resting on the shoulders, the arms draped over it. Look directly at the floor while you twist at the waist to bring your right arm toward the floor. This will simultaneously draw your left arm toward the ceiling. Now, reverse, bringing your left arm to the floor and your right toward the ceiling. Do this to the count of one on each side. Repeat this ten times on each side; as you progress, increase it by five times when you feel ready for it, until you reach twenty repeats.

VI. Bike Innertube—This one is fun. Take the bicycle innertube and walk to the nearest door that has good, solid doorknobs on both sides. Don't use a doorknob that is loose or fragile. Open the door. Now place your thumb at the latch. Drape the innertube over your thumb, holding it against the latch with your thumb. Now, drape the innertube over the doorknob on each side of the door. Remove your thumb and grasp the end toward the floor in your hands. Pull it snug so that it's settled in over the doorknobs. You've now got an inexpensive exercise tool that would cost you plenty of good money in a store or through a television offer.

With the innertube secured to the doorknobs, you can perform a number of exercises to build your arms.

1. Standing facing the door at the farthest point the innertube reaches, grasp the end in both hands, palms of your hands toward

The Broomstick Twist

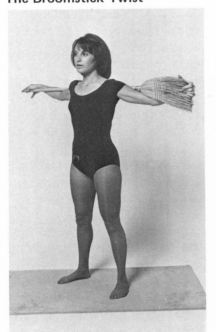
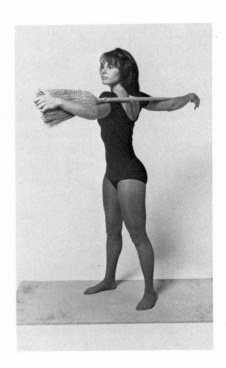

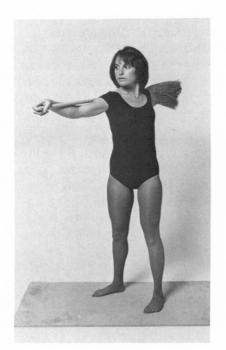

Place the broomstick across your shoulders as though you were an ox with a yoke or a maid in Holland carrying water buckets. Then, similar to the Twist in Chapter 1, twist at the waist, using the broomstick to keep your arms straight and your back vertical.

The Broomstick Bend

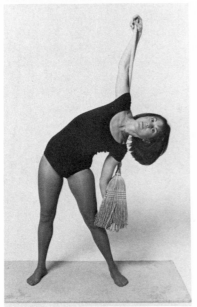

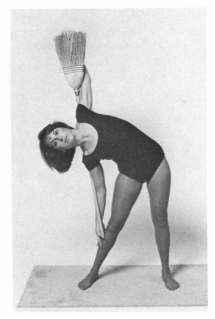

This is similar to the Rocking Chair in Chapter 1, but using the stick.

The stick makes it easier to keep everything straight and on course.

your face. Now, step back one additional foot. Attempt to curl the innertube toward your nose. The innertube, although flexible to some extent, still offers very good resistance. You shouldn't be able to pull it quite as far as your nose. The resistance is what is important. Hold it for a count of two, and then relieve the pressure. Repeat this five times.

2. Now, stand with your back toward the door, at the end of the innertube's reach. The door will pivot a bit to either side to accommodate your use of either your right or left arm. Start with your right arm. Stand as though you were going to put your right thumb in your right ear. Now, slip the innertube into your right hand. Grasp it firmly and attempt to push your arm forward. Hold for a count of two, then let it fall back. Repeat this five times. It's great for the shoulders and upper arms. Do the same with the left arm.

3. From the same position as number 2, drop your right arm to your side, palm forward. Place the innertube in your palm, take a firm grasp, and *gently* attempt to bring the innertube forward, keeping your arm straight. Hold for a count of two, then relax. Repeat that one five times, and then change hands and do it again.

The Broomstick to the Floor

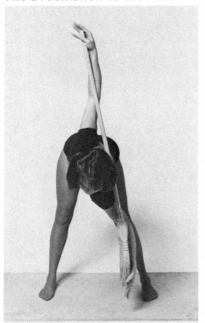

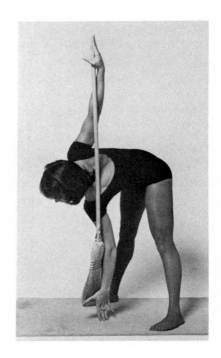

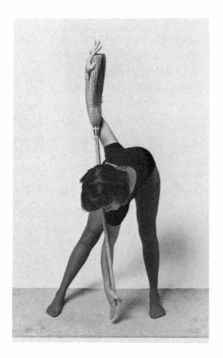

On this one, the difference is that you bend down at the waist, still keeping your legs straight. Look at the floor, keeping your back horizontal with it. Do the alternating twists very smoothly and carefully, making the twists from the hips and not from the back.

Bike Innertube 1

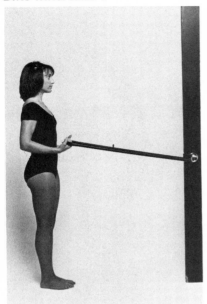

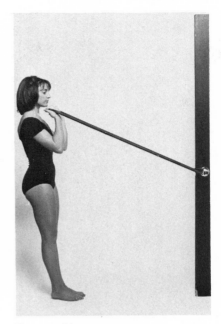

Make sure the innertube is secure.

Try to curl it to your nose.

Bike Innertube 2

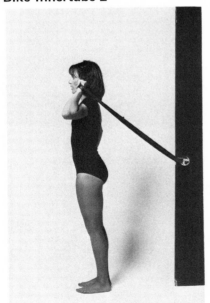

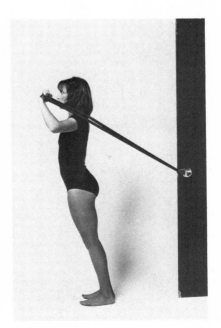

Hold hand at shoulder, and . . .

then try to pick an apple.

Bike Innertube 3

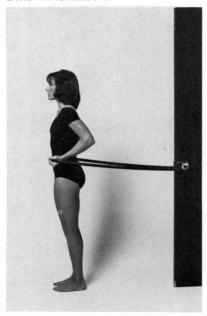 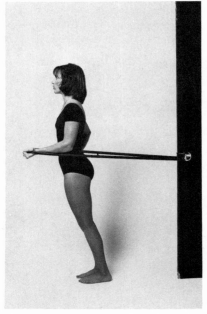

Keep your back straight, and . . .   reach out to shake hands.

Bike Innertube 4

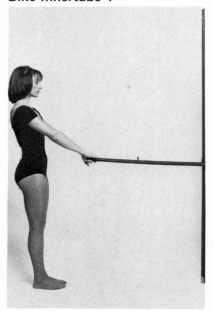 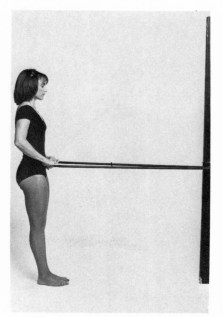

Stand with arms relaxed, and . . .   then pull them toward your hips.

4. Again facing the door, grasp the innertube in both hands, palms downward. Now, walk backwards until the innertube goes taut. Plant your feet firmly, get a good grasp on the innertube, and, with both arms working, try to swing the innertube toward your groin area, working for a count of two. Relax and repeat it five times.

5. Now, come up with some variations of your own on this one. It's fun to make up your own exercises. If you are agile, you can also use the innertube attached to the doorknobs to work your legs, but don't try anything too fancy that will threaten to land you on your posterior. The idea is to use the slight give in the innertube to move to a point of resistance, at which point your holding it for a count will tense and tone the muscles. As you get more comfortable with this, you can hold it for a long count and you can do more repeats.

6. Now, before junior gets home, rush out to the garage and stuff his innertube back into his bicycle tire and pump that sucher up quickly so he won't know you've been using it for something other than a spin around the block.

VII. Bottles of Laundry Detergent—One of the convenient things about gyms and health spas is that they have available a whole truckload of equipment that enables you to work against resistance. By doing fewer repetitions with a heavier object, you can add mass or bulk to an area of your body. By doing more repetitions with less weight, a slimming effect can be obtained. Whether or not you

Laundry Detergent 2

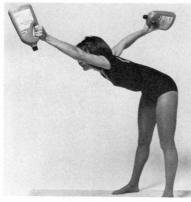

Be careful to do this one carefully.

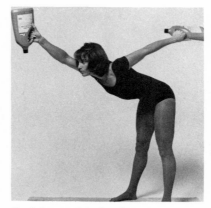

Don't let go of the bottles.

Laundry Detergent 1

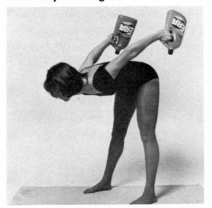

Hold the two bottles firmly, while they rest on the floor, then raise them smoothly behind you (as in photo on left). For Laundry Detergent 3, move the two bottles from center position to left of your left foot, then back to center, then to right, then back to center, repeating the process (as in photos in center). Lying on two chairs, hold the bottles above your head, and then lower them out to your sides, arms straight (as in the bottom two photos).

Laundry Detergent 3

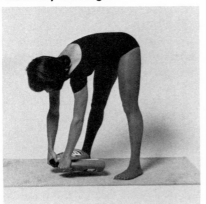 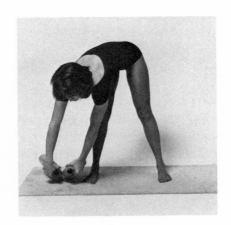

Laundry Detergent 5

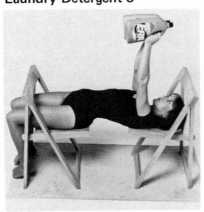 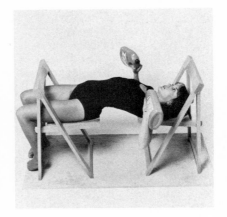

belong to a spa (you may be contemplating joining one), there will be days when you just can't find the time to go by for a workout.

An alternative approach to using their weights would be to keep two containers of liquid laundry detergent available in your bucket. They come in all sizes and you can probably find one that will be the right size for you by hefting it at the supermarket. Purchase the type with handles so they are easier to use. Some of the equivalent weights to contents are as follows:

64 oz. = 4.5 pounds

1 gallon = 10 pounds

Now, haul out your two bottles of detergent (which, by the way, can be used for the laundry in case you forget to keep your regular supply renewed and you run out; make sure that the caps are tightened, so you don't spill the detergent while exercising, because besides getting it on your clothes and the rug, the stuff is in the same price range as gold).

1. Stand with your feet spread apart about twelve to eighteen inches at the base. Holding one container in each hand and keeping your legs straight, bend forward at the waist and let the containers hang in front of you. Move the containers simultaneously toward your back, raising them as high as you can behind you. Hold to the count of two and return them. Don't hesitate at that point, though. Repeat the exercise ten times. This strengthens the arms.

2. Maintain the same position as in the exercise above, bent at the waist, but while raising the right arm back as far as it will go, raise the left arm in front of you. Then, with a smooth swing, reverse it, moving your right arm forward and your left back. All of this should be done fairly quickly, to the count of one. Repeat it ten times. This serves to strengthen and slim the arms.

3. Maintain the same position as in number 2. Now, place both bottles, side by side, near your left foot, while still holding them; be careful not to mash your left foot. Now, move them to a position in front of you. And then to a position at your right foot. Then return them to the left foot and begin again. Repeat this one ten times.

4. Resume standing. Keep the feet spread at the base. While holding the containers firmly in both hands, raise the right arm over the head, resting the right forearm on the head. With your back straight, stomach and buttocks pulled in, lean to the left and then return to the center ten times. Repeat the entire exercise on the opposite side. The plastic bottles will help you bend a bit more

at the waist and will give you more resistance to work against in returning to your center starting position. This enhances abdominal tone, thereby lessening the inches around the waist.

5. Place two chairs together, face to face. If they're wooden, you might consider padding them with a blanket before placing your towel on them.

Lie down, on your back, between the chairs, your hips on one chair seat and your head resting on the other, with enough space between the chairs to allow your arms to move freely.

While you hold one bottle in each hand, settle yourself in comfortably on both chairs. Now, draw the bottles together until they meet at about eight to ten inches above your chest. Simultaneously, now, draw your flexed arms apart and allow them to drop, in a circular fashion, to your sides to points level with your chest. Return them to the same position eight to ten inches above your chest, again using the circular or arc movements with the arms, until they meet. Repeat ten times. This one is especially good for the biceps.

6. Maintain the same position as in number 4. Now, raise both bottles, one in each hand, until your arms are straight above your head, thumbs touching. Bring the bottles down gently until they rest roughly in the crook of your arm, at a level with your chest. Each should be done to a count of two: up above your chest on the count of one, down to the crook of your arms on the count of two. Repeat this ten times. This one is great for developing the triceps.

7. Hold the bottles out to your sides, while lying on the chairs, keeping your arms straight and parallel to the floor. Hold the bottles out there for a count of twenty. Repeat this one five times.

IN CONCLUSION

It is easy to come up with good, fairly strenuous exercises using common household goods. You needn't get fancy and you needn't spend money on anything that either hasn't been used before in some other capacity (the bicycle innertube) or that can't be used in an emergency (the liquid detergent) or that can't be used when not being incorporated into your exercises (the broom and bucket). The use of household items does not have to end with these simple exercises outlined, however. Use your imagination to work other household items into your regular exercising routine. The only limits, are the bounds of your ingenuity.

4

Light Work

Back in the days when *True* was one of the foremost men's magazines in the country, sharing the honors with *Argosy, Saga* and *Esquire*, they used to have a cartoonist who always signed himself VIP. Many of his cartoons were take-offs on a few basic situations. Two of the most common were two guys crawling across a burning desert or two guys chained to the wall of a dungeon. In these stark and tragic situations in life—actually, on the brink of death—VIP found humor.

For instance, he might have the two guys crawling across the burning desert, their tracks vanishing back to the horizon, the sun beating down furiously, the one raising his head with his last ounce of strength, a worried and concerned look on his face, and he says: "I just remembered. I left the bath water running."

Or he might have the two guys hanging from the walls of the dungeon, looking very, very unkempt and bewhiskered and ready to give up the ghost, with one looking at the other very weakly, saying: "I feel a draft."

We'll ignore the two guys out in the desert. We were only using them to show that VIP was not tied into one on-going joke. Let's stick with the guys in the dungeon.

In most American jails, there are rules against putting manacles on prisoners and then tacking them to the cold, stone walls, their feet dangling above the cold, damp floor. Such punishments harken days of jails and prisons and dungeons, reminding us of those great Romantic novels: *The Man in the Iron Mask, A Tale of Two Cities, The Count of Monte Cristo, The Prisoner of Zenda.* These are all tales of heroic noblemen caught in the misfortunes of changing political climates in their countries, thrown into the deepest depths of gristly prisons, and there forgotten for many years, where they make friends with rodents that infest the prison, feeding a rat some of their own bread crumbs, not knowing that the rat's got the same deal with every prisoner in the place and that it's snatching enough crumbs to make several loaves while the poor, kind-hearted, misguided and lonely noble prisoner is virtually starving to death. The prisoners spend their lonely hours watching a spider spinning a web, trying over and over to get it right, failing time after time, but still persevering, only to finally succeed, inspiring the prisoner to write a poem on the lessons learned from the little arachnid. And every prisoner takes time to scratch a notch in the wall each day, to keep track of the passing years.

Now let's face it, the old prisons were far from enlightened, very much unlike they are today, right? Or at least as they are in some countries. In the good old days they threw you into prison and that was it. No one knew you were there and they didn't care. You never got time to stretch your legs in the exercise yards or work in the laundry or have a library card or take a shower or complain about having cooked carrots twice in one week.

Imagine that you are one of those prisoners. You get to sleep all you want. Too much sleep can become boring; but, at the same time, sleep is therapeutic when a person is stressed, so let's say you sleep eight hours out of biological needs and two hours to relieve stress that your body builds up in a day. That's ten hours. Let's say you talk to your rat for an hour, during mealtime; which gives us eleven hours. Then, let's say you are very artistic about how you scratch your daily notch into the wall, and it takes an hour, which puts you at twelve hours. Then, since you're a very reflective person, you watch the little spider three hours a day and find it very entertaining—that's fifteen hours. Maybe two hours of posing for VIP cartoons (after all, how long can you hang suspended from wrist manacles at one session, right?), which brings you to seventeen hours.

That leaves you with seven perfectly good hours.

Let's say that you are the type of person who lives in hope, so you feel certain, especially since the book being written about you is being done during the Romantic era, that you will ultimately—in ten or fifteen years—be sprung from prison. You don't want to come out of prison looking like a scarecrow or a skeleton, because as Romantic novels go, you might have to quickly ascend to the throne or engage in a furious and well-choreographed sword-fight, and you can't do that if you're too weak to lift a scepter or a sword. So what do you do for those remaining seven hours a day?

You could certainly spare at least an hour to exercise, couldn't you?

With no political intrigue and no grand balls and sitting-room small talk to monopolize your time, you could conceivably come out of the dungeon in better shape than when you went in.

But there's a basic problem, isn't there? Since this is the middle of the nineteenth century, they haven't invented the treadmill yet, and if they had, your rat friend would probably claim it for his own; rodents seem to like treadmills. The bicycle hasn't yet been invented, much less an exercise bicycle. And people are still wearing high-buckle shoes; the sophisticated running shoe is still one hundred twenty years in the future. So, confined to a dingy little cell, what are you going to do to stay in shape?

Glad you asked.

Two of the most basic, and perhaps best, places to exercise are on the floor and against a wall, and you've got one floor and four walls all to yourself. You also have a crude plank as a bed and a rough-hewn stool. It's like having a whole gym of your own. And it's so private, you don't even need a locker in which to secure your possessions.

One's home is, of course, much more comfortable and elaborate than a dungeon cell. It therefore offers infinitely more possibilities than that little cell. There are chairs and sofas and archways and doors (that can be opened from the inside) and all kinds of basic, but effective, exercise apparatus around the house—and much of it doesn't even have to be moved.

As a prisoner in the dungeon, you would have been able to stay in relatively good shape; as master of your own castle, the possibilities are almost endless.

Without spending a penny on equipment and without leaving the house, let's get into a sequence of exercises that can free you from the bonds of physical stagnation. It might inspire VIP to a whole new series of cartoons.

YOUR HOME IS YOUR SPA

A good health club, gym or spa can be a real service to your attempts to become and then to keep fit. Unfortunately, health clubs are built on the theory that people have the best of intentions to get fit, but that they'll quickly lose interest. People often find that, after joining the health club, they have difficulty disciplining themselves to find time three or four times a week to visit the club, and it takes three or four serious visits a week to maintain body tone. Unless you are prepared to take full advantage of the health club, it probably is not worth joining.

A health club or spa is not really necessary for exercising. As we are demonstrating, much can be accomplished in the privacy of your own cell...er...home.

Do not embark upon these exercises expecting to do them smoothly and comfortably from the very start. The first few times you try them, concentrate on your form. It's impossible to feel the movement of your body so intimately that you'll know exactly when and if you're aligned properly. If would therefore be to your advantage to do many of your exercises with the benefit of a full-length mirror. Or, if that is impossible, you might consider having a friend act as an observer, helping you get as close as possible to the pictures in the book.

Once you've achieved the proper position for each exercise, concentrate on how your body "feels" in that position so you'll be familiar with it the next time in case neither a full-length mirror nor a friend is available to help. The more familiar and comfortable you come to feel with the exercises, the more enjoyable they'll be.

Do not hold back from doing a good workout, but be careful in reaching your limit and staying on the safe side of that limit. Don't force your body into positions it doesn't want to assume. Be patient and avoid injury. Your ability and flexibility will improve in time. But don't baby yourself; your body is a very flexible, adaptable machine; give it a chance to prove itself.

It is not intended that you perform every one of these exercises in one session. It is recommended that you progress smoothly. Master a few of them first, and then, at the next session, add a few more. The exercises will, in a gradual way, allow your body to adjust to them. We've included quite a few exercises in this chapter, with the hope that you will periodically revise your program by adding or exchanging some of the routines, thereby enabling you to fashion effective yet interesting workouts three or four times a week that do not repeat themselves. This minimizes the monotony factor, which can creep into certain exercise programs. There are many books available with variations on these exercises, and you may want to consult them to customize your workout to your own favorites.

A brief warm-up period should precede any strenuous exercise regimen. Consult previous chapters for proper warm-ups. Don't be bashful about doing your warm-ups and exercises to your favorite music. Exercising should be lively and fun and entertaining.

One note of caution: The following exercises rely heavily upon your floor. If your floor is hardwood or any other hard surface, you will want to place some type of protective padding on it so that you do not injure yourself.

LOTS OF LIGHT STUFF

I. Knee-to-Chest Leg Raise—Lie flat on your back. Extend your arms out to your sides, palms down, to offer support. Keep your legs together. Raise both knees together over your chest, then raise the legs together, your toes reaching for the ceiling, your legs joined. Remember to use your hands and arms to support yourself. Now, again relying on your arms for stability, begin lowering your straightened legs toward the floor slowly, keeping them together, until your heels are about five inches off the floor. Count to five, bring them to your chest again, count to two, and then raise them toward the ceiling. Try to do this one six times, progressing in increments of two every third session until you are doing it ten times. On your last lowering of the legs, try to hold your heels five inches above the floor for a count of ten. If you can't, do as well as you can, remembering patience. Customize this one to your current abilities. This is a great exercise to tighten the abdomen and legs. You'll feel it pulling at some portions of your body that are very much underused.

II. The Cross-Over—Again on the floor, place your hands under your buttocks, palms down, to offer support. Keeping your legs straight and together, elevate them above you as you did in the last exercise. Now, slowly at first, then faster as they become looser, spread your legs as far as they'll go. Now, bring them back toward the center, but instead of stopping there, cross one around the other and keep going, until you again meet resistance. Then, bring them back toward the center, and again overshoot the center, until you are in the spread-leg position again. Now, repeat the exercise, but cross the legs in the opposite way this time. Continue alternating the cross-over. Do six cross-overs with each leg in the first session, increasing it by two every third session, until you reach ten. This one is excellent for the backs of the legs and for the abdomen.

III. The Scissors Kick—Again from a floor position, recline on your left side, resting your head on your left hand, your left elbow on the floor for support. Place your right hand, palm down, on the

The Cross-Over

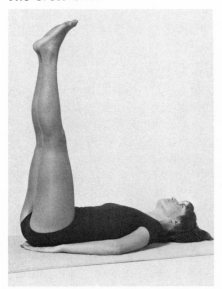

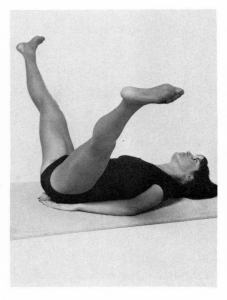

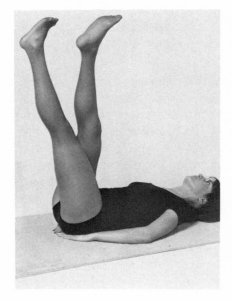

This exercise is excellent for building both flexibility and strength. Lying flat on your back, support yourself with your hands, lifting the legs straight up over the hips, reaching them toward the ceiling. Concentrate on keeping the legs perfectly straight throughout the entire exercise. Spread them into the letter "V". Now, bring them together crossing one over the other, just lightly brushing them. Do not push them too far at the cross-over; just far enough to feel resistance. Then, return them to the "V" position. On the next cross-over, alternate the legs, crossing the one in front of the leg that went behind before. Repeat the exercise, each time alternating the leg that is foremost. Each time that they return to the "V" position, go only as far on the spread as feels comfortable.

The Scissors Kick

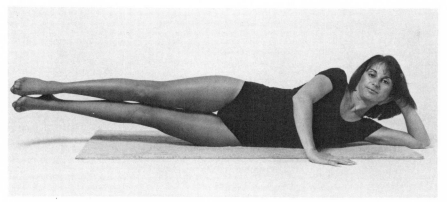

Lie on your side, supporting yourself with one arm, and lift legs together.

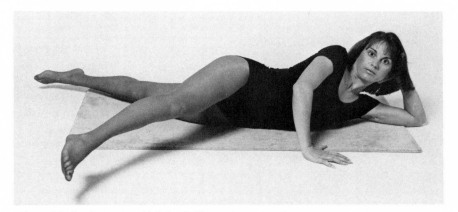

Move right leg forward and left back, like a scissors opening.

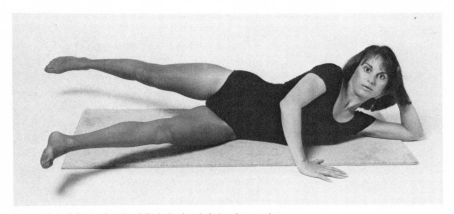

Now, kick right leg back while bringing left leg forward.

Side Leg Raise

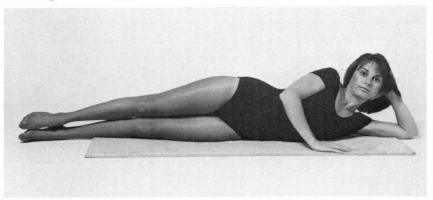

Lie on your side, supporting yourself with one arm, legs on floor.

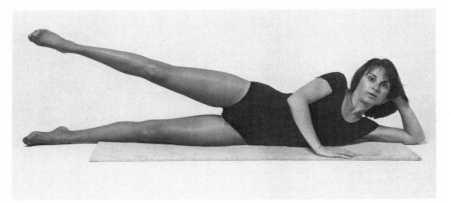

Lift your right leg toward the ceiling, and hold it there.

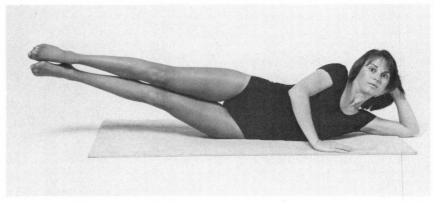

Bring your left leg up to join your right leg; feel muscles pulling.

floor in front of you for added support. Maintain your shoulders, hips and legs in alignment and hold in your stomach. Now, keeping your legs straight, the right above the left, elevate them about four inches from the floor. Bring your right leg forward and your left leg back, as though you were running with straight legs; now quickly and smoothly reverse, using the count of one at each end of the kick. This should be done rapidly and smoothly. Repeat it ten times. Then, turn on your right side and repeat the exercise from that position. This is excellent for the outer portion of the thighs.

IV. The Side Leg Raise Again on the floor, lie on your left side. Again, rest your head in your left hand, your left elbow supporting it on the floor. Keep your body in alignment. Holding your stomach in should be almost second-nature by now. Place the right hand on the floor in front of you for additional balance. Now, raise your right leg about one foot off the floor, keeping it straight. Hold it there as you bring your left leg up to meet it. Continue to suspend it there while you lower your left leg to the floor. Now, return the right leg to the floor. Be careful and attentive as you do this one. There's a tendency to bring the upper leg down while raising the lower one to meet it. There's also a subconscious tendency to lower both legs together. Try to guard against doing either of those things. It is the act of holding that upper leg in the air that brings the best benefits to the inner thighs. Repeat this one ten times on each side.

V. J Kick—This one also begins with you lying on your left side. Start with the same position as numbers III and IV. Slightly flex the lower leg as you tilt your pelvis forward, holding the stomach in. Keep your upper leg straight as you raise it toward the ceiling. Raise it as far as you can without straining; you can allow it to pull a little, but don't hurt yourself. Now, lower it. Raise it again, but this time keep it straight, raise it to the back and up at the same time, and then lower it again, to begin the vertical raise again. Do this one six times initially, increasing it by two times every third session. Repeat it on the other side. It is good for the hamstrings and the buttocks.

VI. Leg/Arm Lift—Lie flat on your stomach with your arms and legs extended, as though you were imitating Superman in flight. Now, spread your hands and feet so they're about eighteen inches apart, measured roughly between your thumbs and your big toes. Here's the challenging part: Simultaneously lift all four extremities, supporting yourself only on your pelvis. Hold this while counting to ten. Repeat it five times. This one is going to be difficult if you've got a stiff back. Be gentle with yourself.

After you've caught your breath, remain on your stomach while grasping your ankles with your hands behind your back. Arch your back and use your arms to help raise your thighs off the floor. Again, you should end up resting on your pelvis. Gently begin to rock back and forth. Concentrate on keeping your back arched. That's the secret. No arch, no rocking motion. As you rock back and forth, attempt to touch your chin to the floor. As you rock backwards, try to bring your chest to as close to an upright position as possible. This one is good for the back, the upper part of the back of the legs, your arms, and your stomach.

J Kick

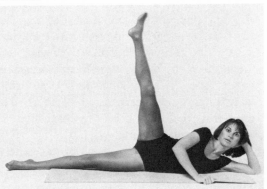

Bring your right leg up as high as you can, keeping it straight.

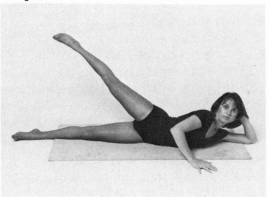

Then, bring it down and back, forming a huge letter "J" in the process.

Leg/Arm Lift

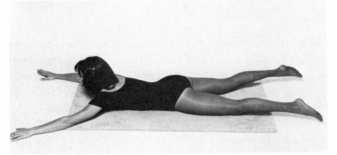

Lie flat on your stomach, as though you were spread-eagled.

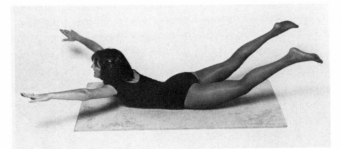

Now, bring your arms and legs about 6-12 inches off the floor.

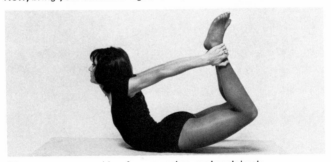

Then, grasp your ankles, form a rocker, and rock back.

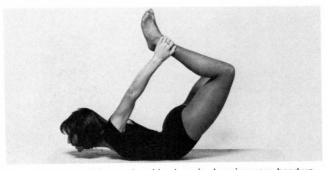

Now rock yourself forward and back again, keeping your head up.

Note: If you have a history of back problems, definitely *do not* do this one.

VII. Quad Stretch—Sit on the floor, bracing yourself by placing your hands on the floor behind you, palms down. Draw your knees to your chest and then spread them apart as far as they will go. Keep your back straight. While keeping the left knee elevated, lower the right knee all the way to the floor, gently touching it to the floor. Now, lower the left knee to the floor while simultaneously bringing the right knee up. Do this to the count of two: lower right knee, *one*; lower left knee, *two*. Repeat this one ten times. Then, lower yourself to your elbows, and repeat the same maneuver ten times. Then, lower yourself to your back, grasp your ankles, and do it ten more times. When finished, attempt to lower both your knees to the floor at the same time. You'll feel this one in your thighs.

Quad Stretch I

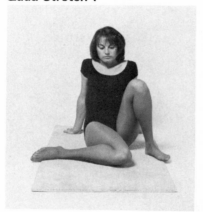
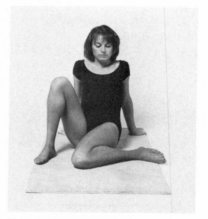

With arms straight and extended, drop your right knee to floor.

Now, bring up the right knee and drop the left knee to floor.

Quad Stretch II

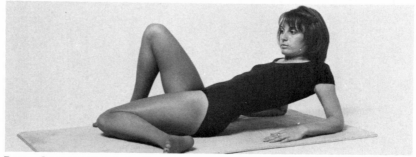

Repeat Quad Stretch I, but with your support coming from elbows.

Quad Stretch III

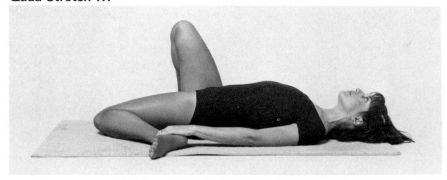

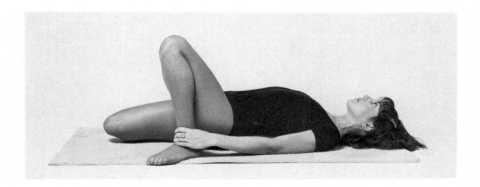

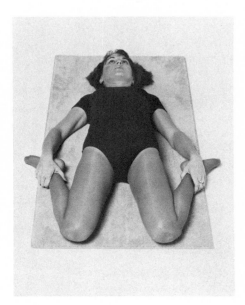

Now, lower yourself to your back and repeat the alternating dip in of the knee with first the right and then the left leg. Feel the stretching in the thighs. Make sure to grasp the ankles firmly. Now, at the conclusion, try to bring both knees to the floor simultaneously; if you are having trouble with that phase, forget it until you become more limber.

The Ham Stretch

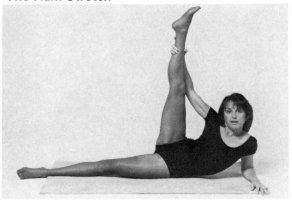

Start by lifting your right leg toward the ceiling, keeping it straight.

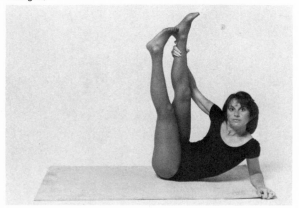

Now, bring your free leg up to join it, support coming from lower arm.

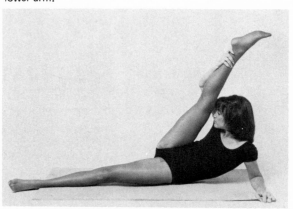

Now, return free leg to floor and ease right leg toward your head.

VIII. The Ham Stretch—Recline on your left side, leaning back on your left elbow for support. Keep your left (bottom) leg straight while you bend your right knee toward your chest, grasping your right ankle with your right hand. Extend your right leg straight toward the ceiling (using your right arm to help), bringing it at a perpendicular angle to the floor. Now comes the hard part. While still maintaining the position of your right leg, raise your left (bottom) leg to meet the right leg, and then lower the left leg while continuing to maintain the position of the right leg. Repeat this process six times. On the final time, after lowering the left leg, bring (with the assistance of your right arm) your right leg toward your nose, attempting to touch your knee to your nose. Concentrate on keeping the bottom leg straight and on the floor. Now repeat the exercise on the opposite side. Every third exercise session, add two more repetitions to this series, until you hit ten.

IX. The Leg: Side-to-Side—Lie flat on your back, extending your arms out to either side with the palms down. Keep your left leg flat on the floor while you raise the right leg straight above you, toes aimed toward the ceiling. Now, on the count of one, move your right leg all the way over to your right side, touching the floor with your toes perpendicular to your backbone. After it touches the floor on the count of one, begin returning your leg to its upright position, passing through that position and heading toward your left, touching the floor on your left side, keeping both legs straight all the time. Once you've touched the floor with your toe, again on the count of one, return your leg to its upright position. Repeat this one ten times. Then plant your right leg on the floor, keeping it straight, and do the same exercise with your left leg, ten times.

X. The Leg: Around-and-In—Lie flat on your back, extending your arms out to either side with the palms down. Bring your left foot up to the bottom of your left buttocks, planting the bottom of your left foot flat on the floor, your left knee bent. Now, keeping your right leg straight, raise it three or four inches off the floor. Make a circle with your right leg, bringing it toward your nose and then looping it out as far as it will go to the right, looping it further back toward its starting position, but always keeping it off the floor. Keep your arc smooth. Do it to the count of one, repeating it ten times. Repeat it with the opposite leg.

XI. The Hovering Pyramid—Lie flat on your back, extending

The Leg: Side to Side

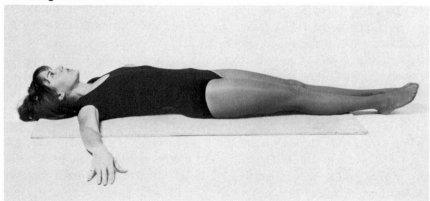

This one is simple. Lie flat on your back, arms out straight to sides.

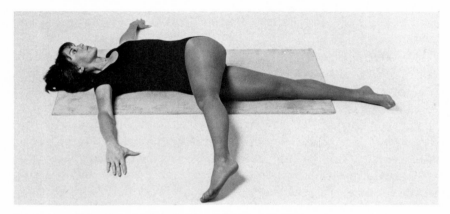

Keeping everything flat except the left leg, roll it over the hips.

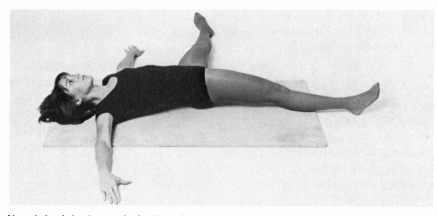

Now, bring it back over the body, and extend it out to the left side.

The Leg: Around-and-In

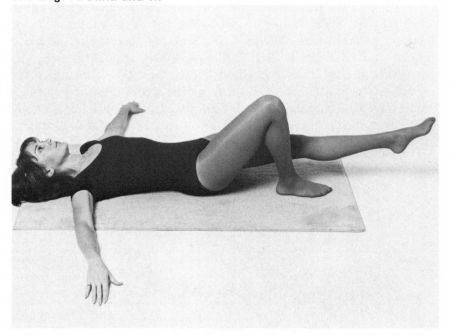

Assume the position of the previous exercise, but bring knee up.

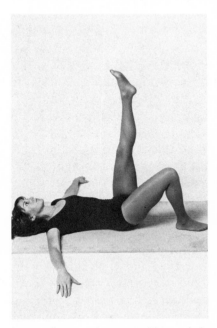

Now, raise your leg up, making a circle, making the loops large.

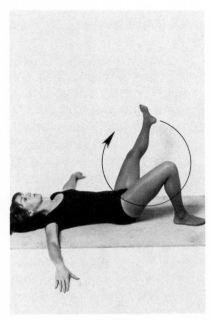

Send the loop out as far to the side as you can. Then use other leg.

your arms out to either side with the palms down. Now, bring both feet toward your buttocks until they touch; plant the soles of both feet firmly on the floor, the heels up against the buttocks. Raise the buttocks as high off the floor as possible, using the thighs, and hold in that position to the count of ten. At ten, relax your buttocks on the floor, keeping the knees bent as your support control. Repeat this one six times initially, increasing by two every third session. This is an excellent exercise for your thighs.

The Hovering Pyramid

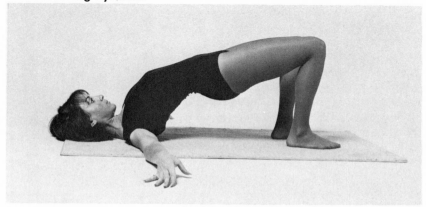

Each week, attempt to raise yourself a bit higher off the floor.

XII. Between the Thighs—Sit on the floor, your back straight, your stomach pulled in, and your legs straight and spread as far apart as they will go. Now, grasp your left ankle with your left hand. With your right hand, make an arch from your right side, up and over your head (keeping your arm straight), aiming toward your left foot, making sure to keep your legs straight all the time. Strive to touch the toes of the left foot with your right hand, keeping everything as straight as possible. While you are stretching for your toes, try to touch your nose to your left kneecap. Bounce twice very gently. Return to center position, then bend forward at the waist, keeping the legs straight, touching your elbows to the floor. Bounce twice gently. Return briefly to the center position, then grasp your right ankle with your right hand, and bring your left hand in an arc over your head and touch your right toes with your left hand, touching your nose to your right kneecap, bouncing twice gently. Do this exercise five times. Finish by grasping your still-spread ankles with the appropriate hands, right hand to right ankle, etc. Now, lean forward, attempting to touch your nose to the floor directly in front of you. Remember to keep your legs as straight as possible while doing this one.

As you progress, add one more repeat of this every third exercise session. Your goal is to get to ten repeats, but don't force your body until it is flexible enough. It is more important to improve the quality of this exercise than the quantity. Concentrate on keeping the legs and back straight, and the stomach pulled in. Don't push this one beyond ten repeats. The exercise is excellent for tightening up the inner portion of your thighs.

XIII. The Bridge—Sit on the floor, your back straight, your stomach pulled in. Draw the sole of the left foot in toward your groin area, resting it flatly against the inner region of your right thigh. Now, bend forward and gently grasp your right ankle with your right hand. As you do this, bring your left arm over your head in an arc, thinking ahead of the arc so that your goal is to touch your right toes with your left fingers. Try to keep your right leg straight while doing this. Now, return your left arm through the same arc, with the left hand ending on the floor behind you on your left. As soon as your left hand touches the floor behind you, use it and your left thigh to raise your left buttocks off the floor while you raise your right arm in an arc over your head, stretching it as far back as is comfortable. Keep the right leg straight while you raise yourself off the floor. Repeat this one five times, then try it with the right leg tucked in toward the left thigh, reversing all the instructions to use the opposite side of the body.

XIV. The Basic Sit-Up—Everyone is familiar with basic sit-ups. You can simplify them in your home by using a heavy chair or sofa that is built with the frame low to the floor. Lie flat on your back, with your knees pulled up in front of you, your feet pushed under the chair or sofa. The toes under the chair or sofa will eliminate the need of having someone there to hold down your feet and ankles when you do the sit-ups; without something to hold them down, they tend to raise off the floor. With your feet under the sofa for leverage, place your hands behind your head with your fingers intertwined. Now, raise yourself to an upright position, doing the lifting with your stomach muscles. As you come up, aim your right elbow to your left knee and touch it. Now, drop down

Between the Thighs

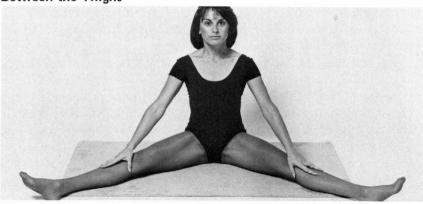

Spread your legs as far apart as is comfortable, back straight.

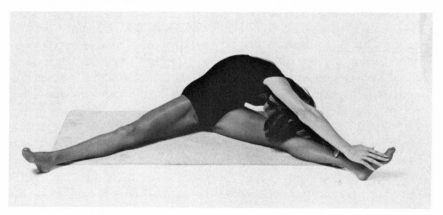

Reach hands toward your left ankle, keeping legs straight.

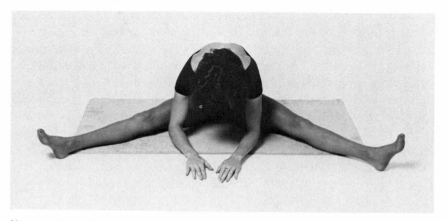

Now, reach arms in front of you as far as you can, bending at waist.

Between the Thighs (cont'd)

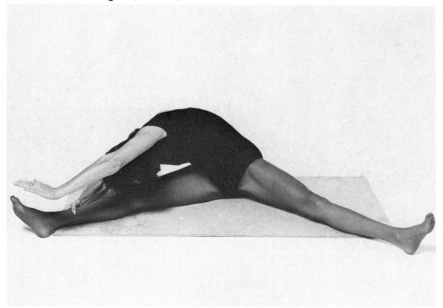

Then, reach the hands toward the right ankle, stretching yourself.

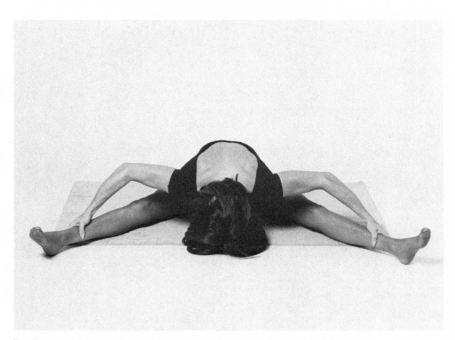

Finally, grasp both ankles, and lower yourself forward, head to floor.

The Bridge

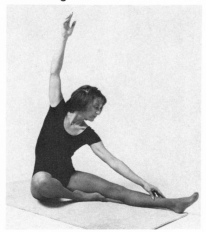

This is a relatively easy one, because you can do it by stretching only as far as you can comfortably. Start with your right sole in against your inner thigh, left hand to left ankle, right hand skyward. Then, reach right hand to right toes. Then, reach right arm over head and onto floor behind you. Finally, raise left arm over head and extend yourself until you feel your entire left side stretch.

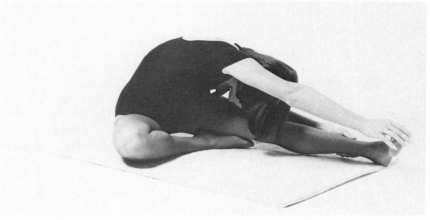

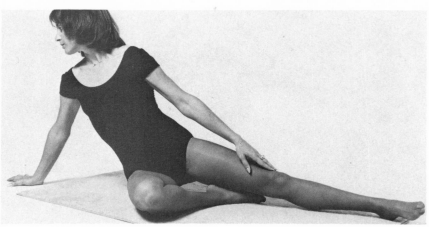

The Bridge (cont'd)

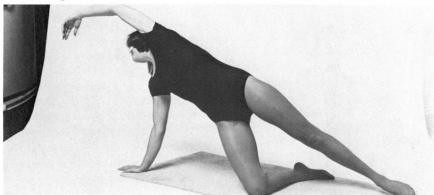

The Basic Sit Up

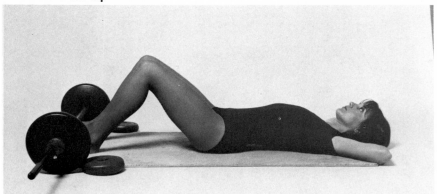

Wedge your ankles under something solid while lying flat on back.

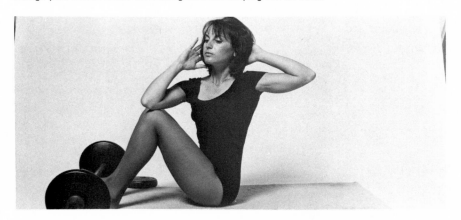

Now, with hands behind head, raise yourself to touch elbow to knee.

The Pendulum

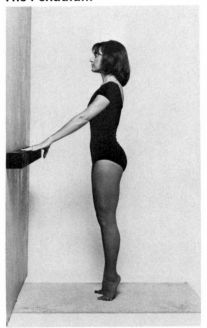

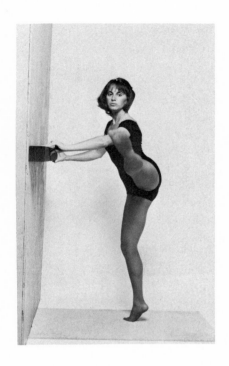

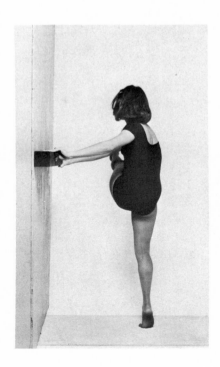

Stand facing a countertop and, standing straight, raise yourself up on your toes. Then, raise your left leg out to your left, keeping it straight. Now, like a pendulum, swing it through (using your hips as the fulcrum) to your right. Keep it up. Now, do the same with your right leg.

and rest your back on the floor. Immediately start your next sit-up, this time aiming your left elbow for your right knee, touching it as you top out. Alternate touching one elbow to the opposite knee. Do six sit-ups the first session. If six is impossible, do what you can. Add one or two more each third session until you reach twenty.

There are variations of the basic sit-up that can make it much more difficult, but we'll ignore those for the time being.

XV. The Pendulum—Rest your hands on either a counter-top or a high-backed chair at arm's length for support. An object about waist-high is perfect. Now, raise yourself up onto your toes. Keep your back straight and your stomach pulled in. Smoothly swing your right leg out to the right as far as it will comfortably go, and when it hits that point, like a pendulum, swing it back to center, continuing it on to the left extreme. Do this one ten times, then repeat with the left leg.

XVI. The Ballet Stretch—Position yourself in front of something supportive that is waist-high, just as you did in number XV. Make sure that you are using something that is heavy and stable. With your left foot planted firmly on the floor at arm's length away from the object, raise your right leg and, keeping it straight, place your foot and ankle on the object. Now, raise both arms straight above your head, your back straight and your stomach pulled in. Concentrating on your balance, bend at the waist, touching your hands to the floor. Bounce twice very gently. Return to a position with your hands straight above your head. Now, bend to the right, over the extended right leg, to touch your fingers to your right toes. Bounce twice and return. Concentrate on your balance and keep your legs and back straight. Repeat this five times on each side, then reverse legs and repeat it five times again.

XVII. The Leg: Back Lift—Stand facing a wall, your toes about eighteen inches away. Now, soles of the feet flat on the floor, lean into the wall with your palms supporting you, bringing your upper body as flush with the wall as possible. Keep your left leg straight to offer support. Raise your right leg behind you, keeping it straight, as far as it will go. Bounce upwards like that ten times, then do it with the other leg. Next week, try it fifteen times. This is a very good excercise for the upper back portion of the legs, the buttocks and those "love handles" around the waist and the upper thighs.

The Ballet Stretch

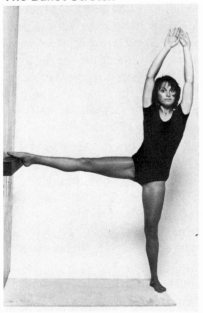

This one is a bit more difficult; leg up on counter, put hands above head.

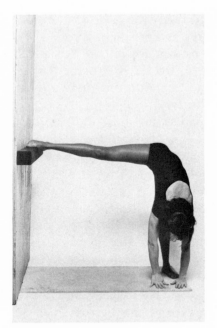

Lower your hands to the floor in front of you, keeping legs straight.

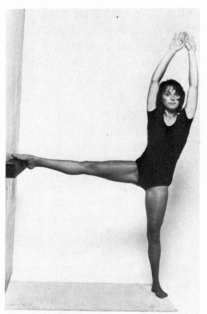

Raise yourself up to the position with hands raised above the head.

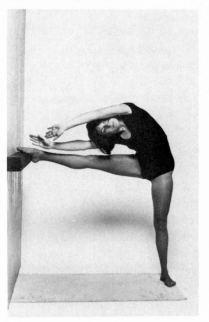

Now, reach in with your hands toward your raised leg, keeping both legs straight.

The Leg: Back Lift

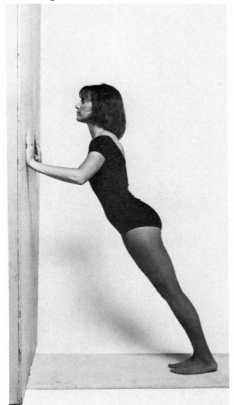

Support yourself against the wall with your palms. Bring your upper body as close to the wall as it can come. The left leg should be straight, sole of the foot planted flat on the floor. Raise your right leg behind you, keeping it straight, until you can't raise it any higher. Then, bounce upwards. Alternate legs.

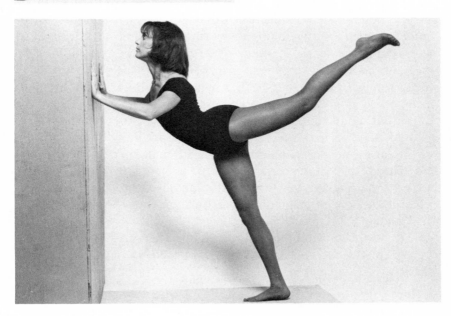

The Invisible Chair

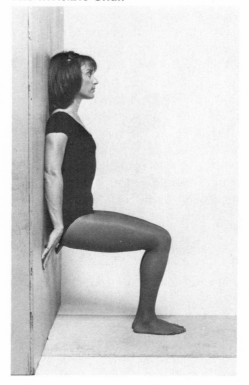

This one is great for tightening up the legs. Stand against the wall, your back pressing against it. Now, slide down the wall by "walking" your legs out from under you, until your thighs are parallel with the floor and your lower legs perpendicular with it. Hold that position for as long as you can. Feel the pulling in the legs.

XVIII. The Invisible Chair—This is a simple but very effective way to build up the thighs. Walk up to any wall in your house, introduce yourself briefly, and then turn around and back up against it, standing perfectly straight. (You can do the book-on-the-top-of-the-head trick here if you wish.) Now, moving your feet away from the wall, slide your back down the wall, keeping it straight. Stop when your thighs become perpendicular to the wall, making sure that your lower legs are perpendicular to the floor. You should now be in a position so that you look as though you are sitting at attention on a straight-backed chair—except that there's no chair. Hold that position as long as you can. You'll begin to feel the pulling in your legs as the muscles tighten to replace the chair that isn't there. Don't overstrain on this one. When you've had enough, use your hands against the wall to help remove yourself from the position, unless your legs are strong enough that you can get them back under you and raise yourself again. Keep your time in your journal so that you can follow your progress.

XIX. Blood to the Head—Standing on your head, instead of being a party trick, can be a very simple and relaxing exercise. And it is relatively easy, even for a person whose sense of balance is not excellent, if you use your wall for support. Walk up to your favorite wall, remove your shoes (you don't want incriminating scuff marks, right?), and get down on your hands and knees while facing the wall. (You can place a towel on the floor if it's hard.) Now, place your hands palm-down about a foot from the wall and on either side of the spot where your head will rest. Your head and hands will act as a tripod to support you. Now, give yourself a generous boost up and raise your legs to meet the wall behind you. Don't panic. You know you're not going to fall over on your back, because your friendly wall is there to prevent that, right? (If you are nervous about this one, you can wait to try it the first few times until you have someone there to help you.) Once you've mastered this by learning to relax and once you've built up your arms with other exercises (and by carrying all those grocery bags), you might want to try a hand-stand (again, against the wall, of course). Once you're up against the wall, stay there for as long as it's comfortable. The increased flow of blood to your head is refreshing and can serve to clear the head on days that seem particularly confusing and mindless.

Blood to Head

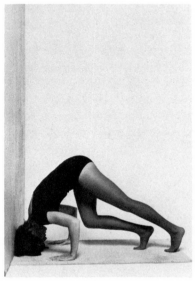

It is a fact that the more blood you get to your head, the better it works.

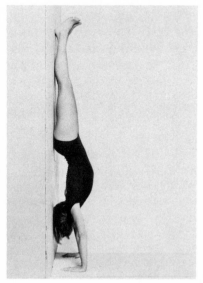

Walk up to the wall, plant your hands, and do a handstand supporting yourself against the wall.

IN CONCLUSION

This chapter is quite an advance from the first three. You must remember not to attempt to do all the exercises in this chapter in one session. Ease into them, adding one or two to your routine at a time. These exercises should be done with some vigor and enthusiasm, and they can be expected to work up a good sweat. That's part of the advantage. Your pores can use that cleansing. And your body can use the work that it's getting. Once mastered, these exercises will prepare you for the next chapter, which is even more vigorous and somewhat more regimented—but also of increased benefit to you. Always remember to follow your warm-up processes (way back in chapter one) before getting into your really serious exercising. Don't race a cold engine.

5

Your Most Important Ten Minutes

Ask five different people what the "top ten minutes of the day" are and you'll get five different answers:

"The ten minutes before the alarm clock goes off in the morning."

"The first ten minutes of lunch."

"The ten minutes before the kids come home from school."

"The last ten minutes of my favorite soap opera."

"I can't talk about those ten minutes in public...!"

For some people it might be ten minutes soaking in a hot tub; or ten minutes of back-rub from a spouse or lover; or ten minutes of peace and quiet that comes unexpectedly; or a ten minute walk around the block in the cool of the evening. For someone who enjoys Western novels, it might be the ten minutes it takes to read the shoot-out scene between the sheriff and the bad guy. For a woman who likes to go to the beauty parlor, it might be the ten minutes it takes to get a shampoo while she lies back and lets the beautician do all the work. To someone else it might be the ten minutes it takes to solve a particularly difficult problem in a class assignment.

Our contention is that we can help you come up with ten minutes in your day that you'll ultimately feel are the ten most important minutes in your daily life.

Ten minutes constitutes only 1/144th of a day. When considered in that context, ten minutes is not very much time. It's one-third of your average situation comedy on television. It's about one-tenth of your average feature film. It's the time it would take a person, walking at a brisk pace, to cover about a half-mile. It equals about forty winks.

What can you do in ten minutes that can make you appreciate, anticipate, cherish, and long for that interim of time?

Our contention is that in ten minutes of your day, you can, over a period of time, tone your muscles and become more flexible and supple, make yourself feel better, appear younger, and become more vigorous.

We could be very sensational about this and make incredible claims for what ten minutes of a day with this program can do for you. But then we'd be falling into the absurd claims many of the highly-advertised rip-off programs are extolling. So let's put it flat out:

Ten minutes with this program will not turn you into a different person. It will not change the color of your hair, cure warts (well, that might not be entirely true, since warts are somewhat caused by your mental health and fitness can improve mental health), make you taller, change the date of your birth, or take the yellow off your kitchen floor.

It promises nothing magic and it gives nothing free.

But the beautiful thing is that whatever it does, it does because you do it. Therefore, whatever good comes from these ten minutes you don't have to credit to a dumb old book. You can take absolute credit for your progress.

You want to feel that the program you are about to embark upon is going to give you some wonderful results, right? You want to be assured that marvelous things are going to happen to you. Well, we can extend certain promises of good things to come if you follow this ten minute program for the rest of your life.

These are ten things that *can* happen to you:

1. You can conceivably, with this and additional programs, lower your blood pressure and pulse rate.

2. You can improve your ability to enjoy life by becoming more alert and energetic.

3. You can increase your ability to participate in sports and recreation.

4. You can increase your ability to participate more thoroughly in love-making.

5. You can relieve at least some of the tensions that beset the average person during the average day.

6. You can prepare yourself for participation in more strenuous aerobic leisure-time activities.

7. You can begin to shift your emotional profile away from periods of depression.

8. You can establish self-esteem and confidence.

9. You can slow the physical and emotional characteristics of aging.

10. You can look in the mirror once a day, and say to yourself, "I'm a better person, physically, than I've ever been in my life, because I'm more able to participate in life now than I ever was before, and I wouldn't trade what I am today for being eighteen years old again."

We could spend some time right now by explaining how each of these ten things can happen to you when you embark on a program of exercise and fitness, but many of them will become apparent to you as the book goes on, and some of them have been expounded upon in various other chapters.

Let's concentrate on getting you started on turning ten minutes of your day into the most important ten minutes out of your twenty-four hours.

This chapter is based on the theory of "The quick brown fox jumped over the lazy dog."

That sentence is one that we learned years ago when we were learning to type. It is a sentence that one types over and over and over again for practice, while not looking at the typewriter keys, because it uses every letter in the alphabet, so that every letter key on the typewriter comes into use—and therefore is imprinted on a subconscious level, so that you'll never again have to look at the keys to find the letters as long as you live. If you repeat that exercise about one hundred million times, you'll be assured of deep knowledge of typewriter keys. It actually works. Some of us took only one semester of typing, spending an hour a day typing things like that silly sentence, just to learn the keyboard. At that point they graduated us to typewriters without letters imprinted on the keys. So sure of ourselves were we, that we stayed up at night making little letters that we could quickly tape to the keys before the teacher came into class the next day.

This chapter features ten minutes worth of exercises that are designed to use, at least passingly, every possible muscle in your body. (You'll notice that there are no exercises for the face muscles; your protestations at doing some of these exercises the first few times will be sufficient to contort your face muscles to the point of exercising them sufficiently. Only joking...)

The exercises are not difficult if you've progressed to this chapter after becoming intimate with the previous four chapters. They should not be repeated too many times at first. And you should not push yourself beyond the point of stress and into the area of pain. The purpose is to stress the muscles so that, like a rubber band, they come back (with some added tension); the object is not to stress the muscles to the point where they are strained.

You may become acquainted with some muscles you didn't know existed; this is because a person, in his or her daily life, usually performs many of the same functions over and over and over. Our lives, therefore, do not call for us to use certain muscles, and therefore those muscles lead a life of benign neglect. Some of them will be surprised that they have been remembered and may wire you, through the communications system of the body, in protest. They're on semi-permanent vacation and they weren't expected back. Reel them in so they can rejoin the rest of your body.

You may ultimately want to extend these exercises to more and more repetitions, and more repetitions take more and more time, so you'll go over the ten minute limit. That's just fine, as long as you are comfortable with it, and as long as you don't come back and say, "Well, you said it would take only ten minutes."

We've checked and timed these exercises, and if you follow them strictly according to instructions, they'll take exactly ten minutes—once you know them by heart and don't have to keep turning the pages of the book to remind yourself how to do exercise number VII, or how many times to repeat exercise number IV.

Do them in a relaxed manner, smoothly, and with a smile on your face. The smile will take care of some of those face muscles that you often forget about during the day. Smile and read on.....

GOING FOR IT

The exercises we're about to run through are technically no more difficult than those in the preceding chapters. Some, in fact, are easier. What makes them a challenging and particularly effective workout is the fact that they are to be performed quickly and non-stop! Strength and flexibility are tested and rewarded, and endurance plays a large part in these. You'll work up a healthy sweat and build up your cardiovascular stamina. *Do not* expect to be able to do these in ten minutes the first time; as you become more familiar—and comfortable—with each exercise, they will begin blending into a smooth routine. If it takes twenty minutes to do them at first, that's o.k. You'll be surprised at how your body will adapt to these exercises. But don't become obsessed with the ten minute goal.

This routine is excellent preparation for the winter ski season, or the summer water-skiing season. You won't suffer with the overall body (and especially the leg) discomfort that usually accompanies those first few days on the slopes, side-stepping mountains, skiing longer than you probably should have on that first time out, and picking yourself up when/if you fall (which, of course, no one in this audience does).

As we've already said, these exercises should be done quickly and with vigor. Doing them to music that has a fast, strong, four-beat rhythm not only helps keep you moving, but makes the workout more enjoyable. The first cut on Boz Scaggs' "Middle Man" LP seems to work particularly well.

This is very important: A warm-up of some type is a must before you begin. Your body needs—and deserves—some general loosening up and stretching before you push it through this sequence.

THOSE HIGHLY PRODUCTIVE TEN MINUTES

I. The Long Reach—With your feet planted about two feet apart, your legs straight, your back straight and your stomach in, raise your arms above your head and loosely join your hands. Turn to the left, at your waist, and keep your legs straight while you place your hands in front of your left foot. Once you've touched there, move your hands to a position in front of you on the floor. Then, move them to touch your right foot. These should all be accomplished in a bouncing manner. While turned toward the right, raise yourself to your standing position, your arms again going above your head. In one continuous motion, turn to your left and repeat the exercise a total of ten times.

When you have finished the ten, with your arms still above your head, begin to bend forward at your waist and, with your legs still straight, touch the floor in front of you, again directly between your still-spread legs, and then stretch to reach behind you. Do this to a count of one. Repeat ten times, moving swiftly and smoothly.

This is helpful to your waist, hamstrings and back. Any exercise that encourages you to hold in your abdomen (and most of these do) also promotes additional abdominal tone.

II. Thigh Work—Stand with your legs apart some three or four feet; lean back into a squat. Tuck in your buttocks. Place your hands on your hips. Now, with your back straight and your abdomen

The Long Reach

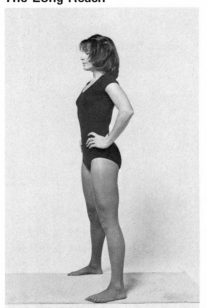

Stand, legs 18 inches apart, hands on hips, back straight.

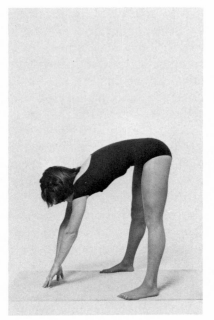

Then, reach your hands on the floor out in front of you, as far as possible.

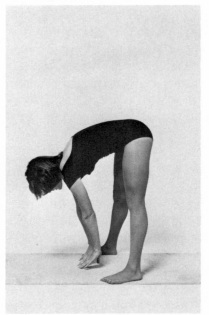

Now, bring your hands out to the floor below your upper body, touching floor.

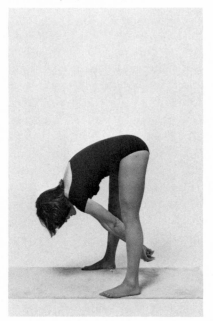

Bending at waist, try to reach your hands as far between legs as possible.

held in, bounce gently four times, going as low as you can. You should feel the pulling in your thighs. Now, redirect your weight from the center to over your left foot, keeping your right leg straight, and bounce four times there. Return to the center and bounce four more times. Then shift your weight to the right foot and bounce four times. Repeat this entire process three times. Then, in a continuous manner, do the routine three times with three bounces, then twice with two bounces, and finally, twice with one bounce.

This will strengthen the front and inner part of your thighs in addition to toning the abdomen. It is also great for tightening the buttocks.

III. Mule Kick—Kneel on the floor on all fours. (Remember to put some sort of padding down on the floor so that you can do these exercises on a soft surface.) Keep your arms straight. Bring your head towards your chest, resting your chin on your chest while you bring your right knee to your forehead. Then arch your back while you extend the right leg behind you, straightening it. Repeat this ten times. With the leg still extended to maximum following your tenth extension, bounce it up toward the ceiling ten times. Then; continuing to hold the leg at maximum extension, lower your upper body to the floor and do five push-ups. Now, repeat the entire process with the left leg.

This is good for the front and back of the thigh. The exercise also serves to tighten the back portion of the hip. It increases flexibility of your neck and back, and also strengthens the arms.

IV. Lateral Leg Extension—Remain on all fours. Extend your right leg to the back, keeping it parallel with the floor. Keep your foot flexed, your toes pointing behind you, and your arms straight. Try to remain perfectly centered and balanced, and do not lean to either side. Now, swing the extended right leg to the right side, parallel to the floor. Turn your head to the right simultaneously to view it as it comes around. Now, swing it back and to the left as far as you can, turning simultaneously to the left to view its approach. Repeat this ten times. Then, with the leg still extended to the rear, bounce it up toward the ceiling four times, and then bounce it forward four times. Repeat the entire exercise on the other side.

This one is geared toward tightening the outer and inner portion of the thigh. It also tightens up the waistline.

V. Frog Leg—While you are still in that position on the floor,

Thigh Work

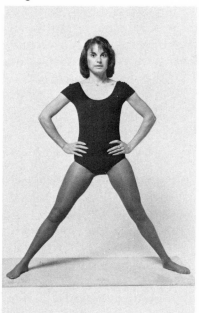

Great one for the upper legs. Stand with legs apart, arms on hips.

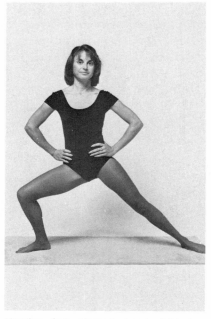

Keeping feet planted, bend right leg, leaning your weight onto it.

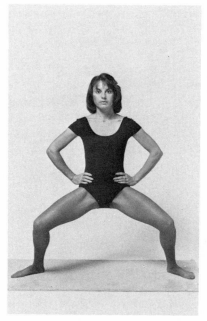

Come back to center, bending both legs at once in a semi-crouch.

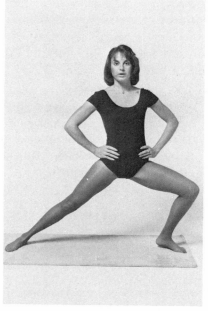

Now, lean into the left leg, keeping the right leg straight.

Mule Kick

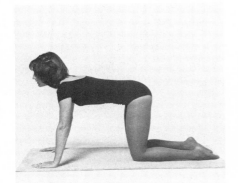

Get into a position of all four on the floor, back straight.

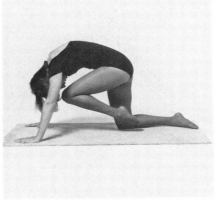

Lowering the head to the chest, bring your left knee to your nose.

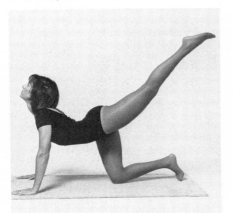

Now, bring up head and throw back your left leg, reaching high.

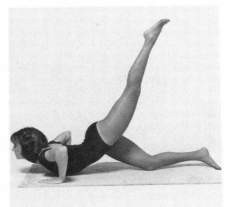

With leg still in air, lower your chest to the floor, slowly.

Frog Leg

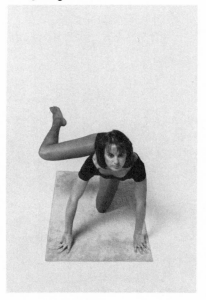

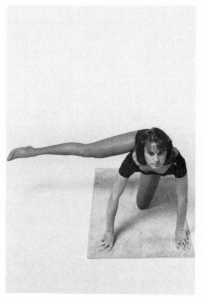

On hands and knees, lift right leg, bring-ing it parallel to floor.

Now, thrust it outward, as though you were swimming, keeping it straight.

swing your bent right leg up toward your side until it gets to hip-lev-el, not too unlike a dog approaching a fire hydrant. You should have your head up and face forward. Your back should be straight. Flex your foot backwards and position your ankle just slightly lower than your knee. Now, extend your leg out to the side and bring it back ten times, like a one-sided view of a frog paddling around the local pond. Repeat this one on the other side so the frog doesn't develop only one side and begin swimming in circles.

This is good for strengthening your back and the outer portion of your thighs and hips.

VI. The Fully-Flexible Leg—Still on all fours, still with your head up and looking straight ahead, extend your right leg to the right side, straight out there, at right angles to your body; flex your foot so that its toes face forward. Your leg should resemble the right wing on a jet fighter plane, with a small fuel tank attached to the wing tip. Lower your leg to the floor and raise it back into position ten times. Then, with your leg still extended, make a small circle four times. Stop and do the same thing four more times but circle your leg in the opposite direction. Repeat this one with the other leg.

The circles make this exercise particularly good for the thighs.

VII. Getting a Leg Up—Still on your hands and knees, extend your right leg to the right side. Keep your head up, face forward. Keep your palms flat on the floor. Now, sit back onto your left heel and return to your kneeling position, keeping the right leg extended and not touching the floor. Do this five times on each side.

We don't have to tell you what this one is good for. You'll know when you give it a try. After such hard work, you deserve a few seconds of what we'll call a rest stretch, because by now your muscles might be threatening to tense up in retaliation for what you're making them do.

Rest Stretch: Briefly, stretch both arms out on the floor in front of you, tuck your head in to your chest and sit back on your heels. Take a few deep breaths and let's move on....

VIII. Leg Pump—Lie on your left side, resting on your forearm. Your left leg should be slightly bent. Swing your right leg, the toes pointed, back and forth ten times, touching the floor as far in front of and behind you as you can. Then bounce/swing your right leg back behind you ten times, keeping it straight. Reverse sides, and repeat it ten times with the other side.

This one is good for the outer and inner thigh and the upper back portion of your leg and hip.

IX. Graduated Leg Raises—Lie on your left side, reclining on your elbow and upper arm. Your body should be straight with your shoulder, hip, and knee aligned. Keep your left leg slightly bent. The right leg should have the heel up and the knee facing down. Raise and lower your right leg (with your foot flexed forward) twenty times. Then repeat the exercise fifteen times while resting on your forearm. Conclude by repeating ten times while supporting yourself with your arm straight. Go to the other side and repeat the process.

This is excellent for the entire leg, especially the outer aspect of your thighs, and the back part of your hip where those "love handles" reside. It is also very good for your arms and abdomen.

X. Going Down—This exercise should be done while holding on to the back of a waist-high heavy chair or dresser. Begin on your toes, heels together. You should be standing at a right angle to the chair or dresser, both your hands extended to the side on the piece of furniture to support yourself and offer balance. With your back straight and your abdomen in, sink down halfway, keeping your knees and ankles together. Hold for a count of ten. (Counting to

Fully Flexible Leg

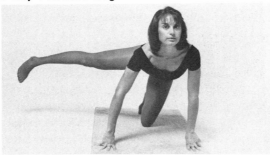

On hands and knees, extend your right leg out, pointing toes to floor.

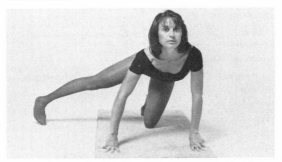

Now, lower leg to the floor and then raise it up again, 10 times.

Getting a Leg Up

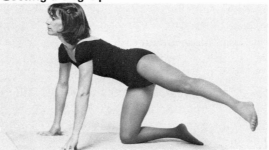

On hands and knees, extend left leg beside you, parallel to floor.

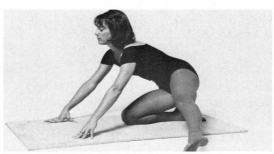

Now, keep the left leg extended while sitting back on right foot; then, resume original position.

Leg Pump

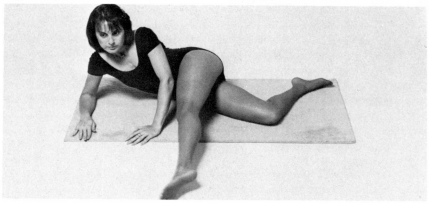

On your left side, supporting yourself on your arm, swing right leg.

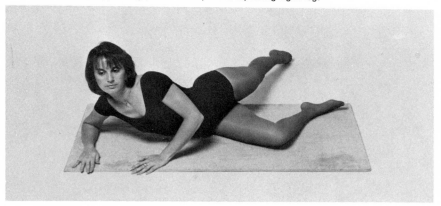

Touch floor as far in front of and behind as possible 10 times.

Graduated Leg Raise

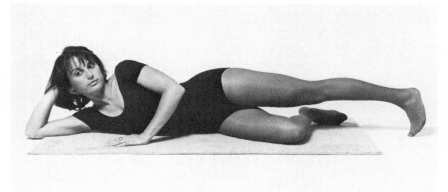

Lie on your right side, reclining on your elbow and upper arm.

Graduated Leg Raise (cont'd)

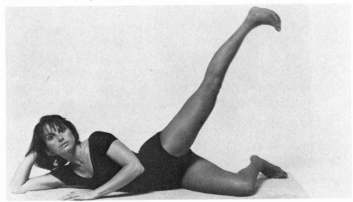

Keep the right leg slightly bent, left leg with heel up and toes down.

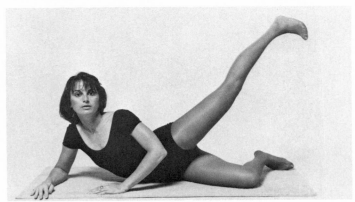

Raise and lower the left leg 20   times, repeating 15 times while on your forearm.

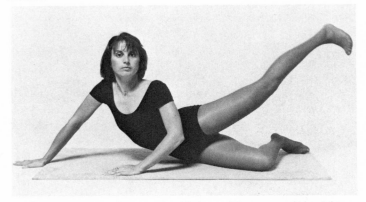

Conclude the sequence by repeating 10 times while your arm is straight.

Going Down

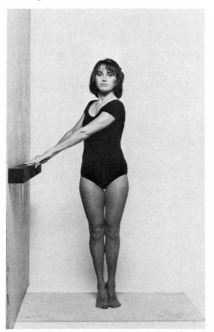

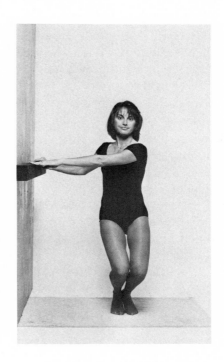

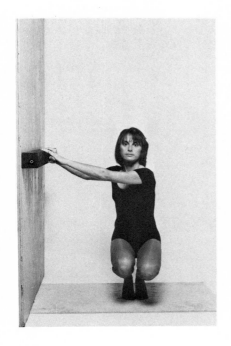

Keeping your heels together, raise yourself up on your toes. Stand at a right angle to the chair, with both hands extended to the side, supporting yourself. With your back straight and stomach tucked in, sink down halfway. Hold for a count of 10, raise yourself back up, and then go halfway down again to the count of 10. (Left) At the conclusion, drop to a squat and bounce 10 times.

ten, by the way, should be the only thing done slowly in these exercises.) Now, come back up, then go down halfway again for another count of ten. Now, drop all the way to your heels and bounce up and down ten times, afterwards returning to a tip-toe position.

This will strengthen your calves and the front portion of your thighs.

XI. Low Work—This exercise is similar to the previous one, but it's done facing the chair or dresser. With your back straight and your abdomen pulled in, begin on your toes and keep your heels together at all times. Again, sink to the halfway position and hold for a count of ten. Now, drop down to your heels and come halfway up again for another count of ten. Drop back down to your heels and bounce ten times. Come up to a standing position and take a deep breath.

This one is specifically for the inner aspects of the thighs.

Low Work

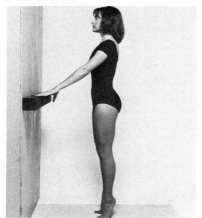

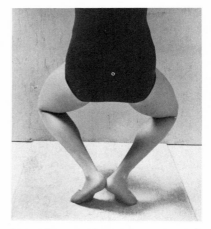

Keep back straight and stomach sucked in, and go up on toes.

Sink halfway, hold for count of 10, raise yourself, drop again for 10 more.

IN CONCLUSION

There, you're finished. Now you can relax and you can be very proud of yourself. You've had quite a workout! Take a few deep breaths and stretch a bit. Then you may want to repeat some of your warm-up exercises to begin cooling yourself off. You've done it. If you can do that sequence four or more times a week, you'll tone up, become more trim and add to your cardiovascular capacity. Congratulations!

exercised that day, the time of day you exercised, where you exercised, and some of your feelings and thoughts following the exercises. It is not uncommon to find that a good, vigorous exercise session clears the mind and produces some unique and interesting thoughts that, if not recorded immediately, are lost forever. The sample journal pages that follow offer a place to jot down whatever is on your mind. There is also space for remarks of a general nature on the day.

At the end of the week's pages, there is a block for reviewing your exercise activities of the week and making some value judgments. How do your muscles and joints feel? How is your energy level? How do these compare with three weeks ago when you started your program? What are your feelings for the week? Do you feel you've made some progress? Do you have a better feeling for your body in general? How has your week gone, besides your exercising?

We've provided a blank set of journal pages that you can Xerox each week and keep together in a loose-leaf book. We've also provided a filled-in set of journal pages to give you an idea how to get started. Some people are reluctant to jot down daily incidents and feelings, while others take to it enthusiastically. It becomes particularly interesting when you go through your first year and then look back at the entries at the start of your journal and compare them with your feelings and fitness at this point.

By filling out and keeping a journal of your progress, you may well be helping some future archaeologists. And who knows, two thousand years from now pages from your journal may be cited on educational television, as some scientist looks back at our era and reverently intones to a breathless audience:

"Energy at week's end was plenty. We can only assume that the people in the 1980s had developed a means of plugging into electrical outlets to recharge themselves, an ability that has—sadly enough—been lost to our modern civilization."

WEEKLY JOURNAL

MONTH _____

SUN. _____

DATE _____

MINUTES OF EXERCISE _____ TIME OF DAY _____

EXERCISED AT ☐HOME ☐WORK ☐GYM _____

FEELINGS & THOUGHTS FOLLOWING EXERCISE: _____

_____

REMARKS ON DAY _____

MONTH _____

MON. _____

DATE _____

MINUTES OF EXERCISE _____ TIME OF DAY _____

EXERCISED AT ☐HOME ☐WORK ☐GYM _____

FEELINGS & THOUGHTS FOLLOWING EXERCISE: _____

_____

REMARKS ON DAY _____

MONTH _____

TUES. _____

DATE _____

MINUTES OF EXERCISE _____ TIME OF DAY _____

EXERCISED AT ☐HOME ☐WORK ☐GYM _____

FEELINGS & THOUGHTS FOLLOWING EXERCISE: _____

_____

REMARKS ON DAY _____

MONTH _____

WED. _____

DATE _____

MINUTES OF EXERCISE _____ TIME OF DAY _____

EXERCISED AT ☐HOME ☐WORK ☐GYM _____

FEELINGS & THOUGHTS FOLLOWING EXERCISE: _____

_____

REMARKS ON DAY _____

MINUTES OF EXERCISE _____ TIME OF DAY _____

MONTH _____

EXERCISED AT ☐HOME ☐WORK ☐GYM _____

FEELINGS & THOUGHTS FOLLOWING EXERCISE: _____

THUR. _____

_____

_____

DATE _____ REMARKS ON DAY _____

_____

MINUTES OF EXERCISE _____ TIME OF DAY _____

MONTH _____

EXERCISED AT ☐HOME ☐WORK ☐GYM _____

FEELINGS & THOUGHTS FOLLOWING EXERCISE: _____

FRI. _____

_____

_____

DATE _____ REMARKS ON DAY _____

_____

MINUTES OF EXERCISE _____ TIME OF DAY _____

MONTH _____

EXERCISED AT ☐HOME ☐WORK ☐GYM _____

FEELINGS & THOUGHTS FOLLOWING EXERCISE: _____

SAT. _____

_____

_____

DATE _____ REMARKS ON DAY _____

_____

TOTAL MINUTES OF EXERCISE: _____

MUSCLES AT WEEK'S END ☐TIGHT ☐RELAXED ☐SORE _____

JOINTS AT WEEK'S END ☐STIFF ☐FLEXIBLE ☐SORE _____

ENERGY AT WEEK'S END ☐NONE ☐AVERAGE ☐PLENTY _____

REMARKS ON THE WEEK: _____

_____
_____
_____

WEEKLY JOURNAL

MONTH *11* **SUN.** **DATE** *16*	MINUTES OF EXERCISE ____ *20* ____ TIME OF DAY *5 P.M.* EXERCISED AT ☒HOME ☐WORK ☐GYM____ FEELINGS & THOUGHTS FOLLOWING EXERCISE: *Stiff from bike ride yesterday. Took 5 minutes to work stiffness out.* REMARKS ON DAY *Beautiful day, no clouds. Went to see Bill race. Day temp in mid-60's.*
MONTH *11* **MON.** **DATE** *17*	MINUTES OF EXERCISE ____ *15* ____ TIME OF DAY *6 P.M.* EXERCISED AT ☒HOME ☐WORK ☐GYM____ FEELINGS & THOUGHTS FOLLOWING EXERCISE: *Felt pretty good. Stiffness gone. Added 15 sit-ups to routine. Went well.* REMARKS ON DAY *Scattered clouds, but pleasant day. Spending day clearing up paper work*
MONTH *11* **TUES.** **DATE** *18*	MINUTES OF EXERCISE ____ *0* ____ TIME OF DAY *0* EXERCISED AT ☐HOME ☐WORK ☐GYM____ FEELINGS & THOUGHTS FOLLOWING EXERCISE: *No time for exercise today. Tried to fit some in after work but got home late.* REMARKS ON DAY *One meeting after the other today. Projects late. Home at 8:30.*
MONTH *11* **WED.** **DATE** *19*	MINUTES OF EXERCISE ____ *25* ____ TIME OF DAY *6 P.M.* EXERCISED AT ☒HOME ☐WORK ☐GYM____ FEELINGS & THOUGHTS FOLLOWING EXERCISE: *very stiff back - probably from the extra sit-ups on Mon. & lay off last nite.* REMARKS ON DAY *More meetings on long term planning - exercise instead of dinner*

MONTH _11_ THUR. _____ DATE _20_	MINUTES OF EXERCISE _15_ TIME OF DAY _7:30 P.M._ EXERCISED AT ☒HOME ☐WORK ☐GYM _____ FEELINGS & THOUGHTS FOLLOWING EXERCISE: _Did some easy sit-ups to gentle back into the routine. Stiff for first 5 minutes._ REMARKS ON DAY _Things seem to be coming together on our schedule at work._
MONTH _11_ FRI. _____ DATE _21_	MINUTES OF EXERCISE _25_ TIME OF DAY _6:00 P.M_ EXERCISED AT ☒HOME ☐WORK ☐GYM _____ FEELINGS & THOUGHTS FOLLOWING EXERCISE: _Added some light exercise to help build upper body. Must add new stuff cautiously._ REMARKS ON DAY _Meeting at 5:00 p.m., went well and quickly. To Mexican rest. for dinner._
MONTH _11_ SAT. _____ DATE _22_	MINUTES OF EXERCISE _0_ TIME OF DAY _0_ EXERCISED AT ☒HOME ☐WORK ☐GYM _____ FEELINGS & THOUGHTS FOLLOWING EXERCISE: _Shoulder stiff from bumping into closet door first thing in A.M. Best to lay off._ REMARKS ON DAY _Left for Hearst Castle at 10:30, late because of dumb accident w/ door. Cloudless day_

TOTAL MINUTES OF EXERCISE: _100_

MUSCLES AT WEEK'S END ☐TIGHT ☐RELAXED ☒SORE _Shoulder hurts_

JOINTS AT WEEK'S END ☐STIFF ☒FLEXIBLE ☐SORE _Feel Flexible_

ENERGY AT WEEK'S END ☐NONE ☒AVERAGE ☐PLENTY _Too many meetings_

REMARKS ON THE WEEK: _Have to learn not to add to many exercises at one time. Must ease into new routines and must stay away from closet doors in the dark. Felt pretty fit on the tour of Hearst Castle, though._

APPENDIX III
SELECTED HARDWARE

Although indoor exercise need not be complicated by the purchase, storage and maintenance of a great deal of machinery, some people seem to gravitate toward such apparatus. Machines can be fascinating partners in a person's indoor exercise program, and we would be the last to discourage a person from exercising—whether with or without machines.

We have surveyed the market and have put together a sampling of the hardware available. We do not claim that the listings that follow are complete. They are, however, ambitious. After surveying the market, we found that at least as far as the more common apparatus goes, there is a great similarity in many models from different companies in like price ranges. We think that what follows will give you a good source of companies working in the indoor apparatus industry, and will also present the spectrum of hardware available.

Most department store chains offer exercising apparatus. Rather than list everything from J.C. Penney to Montgomery Ward, we listed materials available from Sears, because the Sears stores are readily available to most people in this country, they have a good repair follow-up reputation in case your equipment has defects or develops defects, and for people in outlying areas, Sears also has an extensive catalog for those who wish to—or who must—shop by mail.

When shopping for a piece of indoor exercise equipment, take your time checking all alternatives, check prices for servicing and repair, and above all else, try out the equipment in the store before you purchase it and take it home.

Exercise Cycles

Name: Action Cycle (model AC 2)

Manufactured by:
> Walton Manufacturing Company
> 106 Regal Row
> Dallas, Texas 75247
> (214) 637-2500

Price: $339.50

Description: Balanced flywheel maintains smooth coordinated action. Fingertip control adjusts tension to vary degree of exercise. Handlebar and seat synchronized to pedal action. Non-electric. Pedaling activates mechanical unit. Foot straps, large padded seat and chromed handlebar heights are adjustable. Black matte finish on metal parts. Heavy vinyl-clad reinforced steel cover with wood-grain finish. Chain drive mechanism with pre-lubricated oilite or ball bearings at all movements. Features two and one-half to one reduction from pedal revolution to handlebar movement or handlebar and seat movement coordinated action. Weighs sixty-five pounds.

Name: Air-Dyne (model AD 2)

Manufactured by:
> Schwinn Bicycle Company
> 1856 North Kostner Avenue
> Chicago, Illinois 60639

Price: $438.00

Description: A total concept exerciser, for both the upper and lower body. An entirely new air-resistance principle provides a smooth, continuous workload. The entire unit is a sophisticated exerciser permitting a continuous, repeatable work measurement. Workload indicator reading kpm/min., sweep second hand timer, resettable and cumulative odometers, easily adjusted saddle height. Arm levers move to exercise upper body while legs are turning pedals. Weighs seventy-seven pounds.

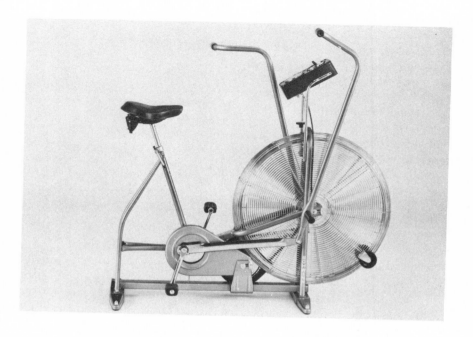

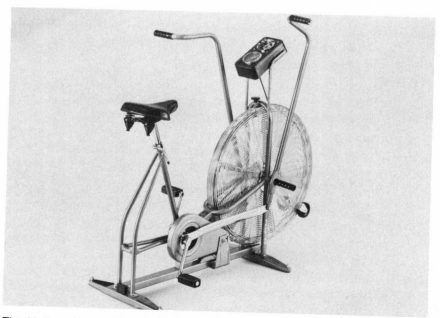

The Air-Dyne is a sophisticated, advanced design on the traditional exercise cycle in that it uses vanes to provide resistance..

Name: Carrousel Jogger (model 616)

Manufactured by:

Walton Manufacturing Company
106 Regal Row
Dallas, Texas 75247
(214) 637-2500

Price: $269.50

Description: Mechanical unit activated by leg action. Balanced steel flywheel maintains momentum of synchronized chain and sprocket mechanism. Use of unit provides lifting and lowering of legs as in running and jogging. Speedometer/ odometer. Twistable handlebar. Chrome-plated legs and handlebar. Weighs fifty-five pounds.

Name: Classic Electric Cycles (model VS)

Manufactured by:

Walton Manufacturing Company
106 Regal Row
Dallas, Texas 75247
(214) 637-2500

Price: $499.50

Description: Adjustable speed control to vary pedal revolutions from thirty-eight to seventy-four rpm. Horseback-like riding and cycling simulates fully automatic units with three-way coordinated action of pedals, handlebar and seat. Powered by a ¼-hp, 120-volt, 60-cycle, high-torque motor. Can be pedaled without using the motor. Pre-lubricated oilite or ball bearings at all movements. Chain and sprockets for drive mechanism with 1.7 to 1 reduction from pedal action to handlebar and seat movement. Foot straps, large padded seat and chromed handlebar heights are adjustable. Black matte finish on metal parts. Heavy vinyl-clad reinforced steel cover with wood-grain finish. Weighs ninety pounds.

Name: Commodore Bike (model 404)

Manufactured by:

Walton Manufacturing Company
106 Regal Row
Dallas, Texas 75247
(214) 637-2500

Price: $139.50

Description: Welded frame construction of one-inch diameter steel tubing. Heavy spoked rim with 20" x 1.75 tire. Quick adjustment for heavy-duty seat and handlebar height. Chain drive and positive fingertip control for accurate setting of resistance to pedaling. Combination speedometer and odometer. Weighs forty pounds.

Name: Contemporary Electric Cycles (model 701 V)

Manufactured by:

Walton Manufacturing Company
106 Regal Row
Dallas, Texas 75247
(214) 637-2500

Price: $539.50

Description: Motorized cycle and rowing action, fully automatic unit with three-way coordinated action of pedals, handlebars and seat. Powered by ¼-hp, 120-volt, 60-cycle, high-torque motor. Can be pedaled without using the motor. Pre-lubricated oilite or ball bearings at all movements. Chain and sprockets for drive mechanism with 1.7 to 1 reduction from pedal action to handlebar and seat movement. Foot straps, large padded seat and chromed handlebar heights are adjustable. Vinyl-coated sheetmetal panels with Danish walnut wood-grain finish. Adjustable speed control to vary pedal revolutions from thirty-eight to seventy-four rpm. Chrome-plated steel frame and legs. Weighs ninety-five pounds.

Name: Deluxe Exerciser (model XR 6)

Manufactured by:

Schwinn Bicycle Company
1856 North Kostner Avenue
Chicago, Illinois 60639

Price: $197.95

Description: Your basic exercise cycle. Saddle and handlebar adjust easily without tools to fit most any rider. Takes up a relatively small space. Built-in pedal resistance control simulates real bicycle riding, of which Schwinn knows a great deal. Sturdy construction with wide base plates for firm footing. Has a reading stand available. Speedometer/odometer, dial-type resistance control and timer. Weighs fifty-six pounds.

6

Heavy Equipment

Ray Bradbury wrote a short story that gave a child's view of an apparatus-laden playground.

To adults, the playground was the pride of the neighborhood. It had all the modern equipment including slidingboards, merry-go-rounds and maypoles.

To the child, however, the playground was like a torture park. Every piece of equipment had some loathesome, painful memory for him. He'd fallen from this, skinned his knee on that, and the spinning and twirling had made him nauseous. His parents couldn't understand why he was so reluctant to go to the playground to have fun.

Many people have a similar response when they walk through the doors of a health spa or gym. Faced with an array of equipment with weights, cables, handles and push pedals going in seemingly a thousand directions, and people grunting, sweating and sometimes swearing, is enough to make the first-time visitor feel he or she has been dropped, unwarned and unprotected, into the middle of a demon's den. This feeling is aggravated by the fact that most modern health spas have mirrors everywhere. Mirrors often make the suffering and exertion and misery in the room overwhelming.

Some people stand petrified in the doorway, take a deep gulp, politely turn around and leave. If you've already signed your contract and paid your money, this is just fine with the spas. They operate on the assumption that a certain (fairly large) percentage of paying customers will never bother showing up to use the place. Or at least they will use the facility infrequently. If everyone who belonged to the local health club or spa arrived at the same time, it would look like the French peasants storming the Bastille.

To many of us, a gym looks like a chamber of terrors. Big, hulking people strut around, examining themselves in the full-length mirrors. They flex here and there, grinning in obvious approval, while their very presence intimidates others who are neophytes to the place.

Before the advent of the plush health centers, weight-lifters and body-builders worked out in dark, either humid and overheated or dark and chilly little weight rooms behind boiler-rooms in the basements of gymnasiums. You'd see them emerging every once in a while, like bears coming out of hibernation. They'd paw the ground and look around as if they were from another planet or perhaps a bit demented; it seemed as though they'd never seen the sun before or as though, no matter how many other people were outside the gym, no one else existed.

For someone new to the weight or workout room of a health spa, even being around those guys can be intimidating. They can be the most soft-spoken, incredibly nice people in the world, but there is always the feeling in the back of your mind that they are so into what they are doing that, after you've waited in line to use one of the pieces of equipment they were working out on, and after you'd lowered yourself into the position to press up some forty or fifty pounds to their one hundred eighty, that they'd come back to the piece of equipment, never even notice that you were there, position themselves in the bench, and begin pushing up one hundred eighty pounds, squashing you into the thickness of a 1957 commemorative stamp.

There is also a feeling of frustration on the part of the neophyte—frustration at not knowing how to use the equipment. Let's face it, some of this stuff looks as though it was designed by a nuclear physicist, with a hundred different settings and a seventy-four page operation. The confusion is usually complicated by the attendant. If you're a guy, the attendant shoves you off to the locker room, telling you to change and come back out here, and he'll get you going on the equipment. When you come out, he's usually smiling and talking very earnestly to one of the female attendants, as though he's trying to get her to occupy a locker with him. (She is merely trying to figure out which locker.) You cough to get his attention, but it seldom works. You inch closer; you hear some of the conversation; you inch away and back into a wall. The smack of your head against the wall reminds the guy of your presence. He looks up with a practiced smile on his face, nods at you, leans down and whispers something entirely humorous into the girl's hair, and slinks over to your side.

He leads you back into the weight room as though he's known you all his life, introduces you briefly to several of the heavies, and whispers conspiratorially to you that so-and-so was a finalist in the Mr. America contest in 1968 and he works out here all the time. Which is supposed to imply, apparently, that if you work out here all the time, you can become a finalist in a Mr. America pageant that was held twelve years ago.

After leading you to one of the pieces of equipment and asking you which brand of muscleman you want to be, he takes your measurements to see how many centuries it's going to take you to make it, writes the information down on a card, and begins explaining the machinery to you. He's done it so many times before, however, that some of the words run together. He might as well have been explaining the insides of a computer or selling you a vacuum cleaner. It all sounds the same. "Okay," he says, "you understand?" You're too embarrassed to admit that you don't, so you nod sheepishly and he smiles at you and walks out to take up where he left off with the female attendant, patting her on the behind as he herds her away to some dark corner of the sauna.

You end up trying to be inconspicuous, hoping someone else will come over to use the piece of equipment so you can watch what they do to get it started. Or else you look for the most simple piece of equipment in the place and gravitate toward it.

Besides a chinning bar, which has been evolutionized into something with two handles that is part of a much more complex structure, the most simple things in the room seem to be the stationary bicycles and the treadmills. After all, almost everyone in the country has a childhood that included a bicycle, and everyone knows someone who had hamsters or herbils that played for hours on a treadmill that was monotonous and squeaky enough to keep them awake all night.

The bicycles seem easy enough, so you give one a try. It has gauges on it, however, which perplex you for a few seconds until you realize that they are a speedometer and an odometer, to tell you how fast you're pedaling, and how far you're going while going nowhere. Some of the bicycles also have another control that takes several forms, often a thing like a doorknob, that, upon turning, will increase tension on the wheel so that it's harder to pump. You have just discovered the exercise cycle.

After working up a sweat there, you wait until the guy who's been jogging on the treadmill gets off and you hop on, while it's still going, which is comparable to stepping out of a car that's going fifteen miles per hour. After breaking your chin on the bar in front of the treadmill, you turn it off, spread your feet on both sides of the belt, and start the belt at a walk. You finally get the hang of it and begin increasing the speed.

It's nice to have a mirror on the wall in front of you so that you can watch your form and so that you'll have something better to look at than a bare wall while you're running to get nowhere. If it's positioned correctly, the mirror will also allow you to see what the male and female attendant are up to without them suspecting—not that they care anyway.

After ten minutes on the treadmill, you dismount, swagger about for a minute or two, and head for the sauna, where you stay for a few minutes until you think it will burn out the lining of your lungs, and then you take a shower and head home, a good day's exercise behind you.

There are some companies that manufacture apparatus for the home, because they realize that some people don't want the hassle of going to a gym. Let's take a look at what the equipment is, how it can be used, its pros and cons (the space it takes up, the noise it can make, and the required maintenance), and some of the ways a person can incorporate this equipment into a daily exercise routine. Some of these can also be terrific for breaking a lease at an apartment.

HARDWARE LOOKS FOR A HOME

Your prime consideration, when contemplating purchasing exercising equipment for the home, should be how that equipment will mesh with your living quarters. (Considerations such as cost, use potential, quality and value, etc. are all secondary, and we'll discuss those aspects shortly.)

A set of dumbbells or a Bullworker can be compatable with virtually every living situation, whether you are currently residing in an apartment complex with walls as thin as twenty-pound bond paper or in a farmhouse with the next human being two miles beyond the hills.

Some of the more sophisticated, weighty equipment, however, does not lend itself to certain living situations.

Some exercise cycles and many treadmills, for instance, are quite noisy. An apartment complex, where people are living in close proximity, is probably the last place on earth that will welcome such equipment. Consider the discomfort to someone either next to or below the apartment with a treadmill that is run perhaps an hour a day. Even in a well-constructed apartment complex, one with good walls and solid floors, the rumble of a treadmill is going to become maddening to the neighbors. It will almost invariably cause vibrations that will be as annoying as hearing a jackhammer tearing up the street.

The solution to putting the treadmill in your apartment might be to set it up in your apartment complex storage area, where you can lock it in your cubicle. Unfortunately, a storage room in the basement of an apartment complex is not a very favorable place to spend an hour of each day. You'll end up with an acute case of claustrophobia.

The ideal situation, of course, is to own a single-family dwelling, preferably with a basement, where the apparatus can be set up out of the mainstream of traffic through the house and where its rumbling will sound like a mere earthquake to people on the first floor of the house. (That is, of course, exaggerating a bit, because some of the newer designs in treadmills are fairly quiet, although they do become noisy when they begin wearing out and when they are in need of maintenance.) If you are in an apartment or condominium complex, it would seem best to forget the heavier equipment, such as exercise bicycles, treadmills, rowing machines, etc. Many of the more modern complexes offer an exercise room that features this type of equipment as part of your rent or condo fees.

If you have a home, and can fit the piece of equipment in some convenient spot, an exercise bicycle or a treadmill might be a very good idea, especially if you have cold, cruel winters that don't invite you outside to get in some of your workouts.

After exploring the possibilities of a good place to house the equipment, or after nixing the idea because there is no such place, the next thing to consider is perhaps the most difficult question: Just how extensively will you make use of that piece of equipment?

If you are completely honest with yourself, you may realize that exercise equipment will gather dust like many other such things you've "invested in." Don't feel embarrassed about that. Much of the business of America is done on the impulse-buying plan. Our storage room in the basement doesn't have space for a treadmill, either, because of things we purchased and have in storage. Anyone interested in buying one of the original Odyssey television games? The games with the little dot that moves around the screen and that does little if anything else? If you feel you'll get your mileage out of an exercise cycle or treadmill (no pun intended), one or the other or both may be a worthwhile investment.

Your next logical step should be to survey the market. (In Appendix II, we have gathered many of the available pieces of indoor exercise hardware, with information on price, manufacturer, etc.) By surveying the market, we do not mean to only read about the equipment; go by a dealer's and try the equipment on for size.

If you're a two hundred-twelve-pound male contemplating purchasing a treadmill, you're going to want to make sure it's a good, sturdy one that is not going to break down every few days under your pounding. Look at the treadmill or exercise cycle or rowing machine as an investment—and investments should be long-term while they're delivering dividends. In this instance, the dividends are the fitness, while the long-term investment is the machinery still being functional after several years of workouts. Expect to pay for longevity. Some of the newer treadmills offer electronic telemetry equipment that will give you a constant read-out of essential functions happening within your body as you exercise on the equipment. That is an option that is not necessary, but, if affordable, can be helpful in regulating your output of effort, so as not to get into a situation where you are straining too hard.

You may want to check with the dealer on the possibilities of purchasing a smaller model at this point, with the option of trading it in on a larger and more sophisticated model if you find that treadmill running is for you. As with anything else you purchase, check out the warranty that comes with the piece of equipment, check into how long (and how costly) it is to have the thing repaired if it breaks down, and you might want to check publications such as *Consumer Reports* for unbiased testing and evaluation of the various machines.

We currently reside in a condominium unit that is on the third floor, and therefore do not have any such equipment. We like to do our running and bicycling on the roads. Of course, we don't get snow where we live, or we might welcome some indoor exercise equipment so we could thumb our noses at the ice and sleet while running on a treadmill in the comfort of our home, going so far as to have stereo headphones on to make the luxury complete.

We prefer to keep our indoor exercising simple, going no farther than the mate:ials in the Bucket Brigade chapter. Friends of ours, living in single-family dwellings, do have exercise cycles which they use while reading or watching television. We've both used treadmills and exercise cycles at health spas, however, and can certainly see their value.

Let's assume, for the sake of argument, that you are considering purchasing one or more pieces of exercise equipment. Let's discuss their uses and their good and bad points.

EXERCISE CYCLES

Cycling is an excellent aerobic exercise—if it is sustained. The continuous effort at a relatively easy rate elevates the functions of the lungs, the heart, the blood vessels, and the leg muscle groups. There is not a great deal of stress or tension placed upon the systems, as long as the cycling is being done on a level surface and as long as it is being done smoothly. Bicycling longer than the body is prepared for will cross the threshold and force the body into anaerobic effort, of course, but that is not where our attention lies in this discussion.

The cycling process, if it is done for an extended period of time, does wonders toward developing the entire cardiovascular system, which contributes to lowering the resting pulse rate, strengthening the heart and making the blood-flow more effective. Eventually, as the body adapts to the work it is being asked to do in the cycling, it can do more and more, going longer and longer. And, consequently, to make the body more fit, one must do either more and more cycling or more difficult (i.e., hill) cycling.

By using the exercise cycle, however, one need not look forward with trepidation to spending hours per day pedaling over hill and dale, facing hostile traffic, hostile dogs, and hostile weather.

Another way to continue becoming more fit once your body has begun to adapt to effort is to add slightly more resistance. The exercise cycle has a control that will apply a growing amount of resistance, so that as you become stronger the exercise cycle will allow you to keep improving.

The benefit of the exercise cycle is that you can do other passive things in your home while you are riding the cycle. It is easy to place the television in front of you so you can watch your favorite program, you can listen to music on the stereo (although you may have to turn it up relatively high to be able to hear it above the whirrrr of the cycle), you can read a book or a newspaper, or turn the cycle to a window and just daydream as you watch the outside world.

The modern exercise cycle is not as loud and noisy as some of the older types. Some of them, in fact, are quite quiet, except for a whirring sound. They are likely to be one of the least offensive of the indoor exercise machines.

If you are going to be serious about mounting and riding the exercise cycle on a regular basis, you will likely perspire freely while using it. It is therefore a good practice to place something (a towel or a mat) under the cycle to absorb the perspiration, because if you let it drip onto a hardwood floor or a carpet, over a period of weeks it will have a devastating effect.

Although it is going nowhere, an exercise cycle used an hour at a time some four or five times a week does experience quite a bit of mechanical fatigue. It is wise, when considering such a purchase, to buy one that is slightly stronger than you anticipate you'll need. It is also imperative that you follow the maintenance instructions, because having it in for repairs several times a year is going to end up costing you more than the original purchase price.

We like to have some idea of how much work we've done when we're finished (we're compulsive about putting our effort down into our journals for posterity and reference), so one of our considerations when purchasing an exercise cycle would be to make sure that the instrumentation is all solidly built and functional. That is, we'd want to have a good speedometer and odometer. We've seen some fairly expensive cycles with really shoddy instrumentation—instrumentation that is easily broken and that regularly leans toward the side of inaccuracy.

If your entire family plans to use the cycle, you can certainly justify a top-of-the-line model. Again, though, if you know yourself well enough to realize that sessions on the exercise cycle are all a passing fad, don't bother purchasing one—drop by a health spa when they have guest passes available and take out your frustrations on theirs. In fact, it would be worth a visit to several health spas to see just what characteristics you want in an exercise cycle. Or, make the rounds of the exercise cycle dealers. Shop for your cycle like you'd shop for a car—and don't be afraid to dicker on the price.

TREADMILLS

Treadmills have always held a connotation two steps left of human—perhaps because they are so often associated with rodent-type animals. The connotation really comes home if you've ever tried to sleep in the same room with a pair of gerbils housed in one of those see-through plastic Habitrail things with the red wheel. After three nights' worth of vigorous running, the wheel squeaks and wobbles, so that it sounds similar to a B-29 that's just taken one too many machinegun bullets in its starboard motor. And gerbils, being the perverse little creatures that they are, seem to take great pleasure in using the wheel for longer periods of time as it becomes noiser. Combine that with the fact that they are nocturnal creatures, and you have perfect-pitch insomnia.

Since rodents having treadmill-running down so well, it seems like a waste of time for human beings to compete with them. But they invariably do, and with a vengeance. (Rich here: People are somewhat like gerbils, I suppose. When I began running after a decade layoff, I was living in Alexandria, Va., and I frequented a health spa in the winter months and used their treadmills. Being very clumsy and very much lacking in good balance, I knew that if I tried to run on the snow or ice, I'd injure myself beyond redemption. I was not, of course, the only person using them. They were seldom at rest. As soon as one person stepped off, there was someone else ready to take over. Sometimes lines formed. As a result, and despite the fact that they were supposed to be industrial strength treadmills, the things were always breaking down. And, the worse they got, the more people tended to use them. I suspect it was a perverse pleasure for the guy who could be on the thing when it finally broke. He could come off the thing, arms raised in victory, and declare: "I did it. I conquered the damned machine." This is a cry that most human beings relish. Unfortunately, the machine did not always lose in a sportsmanlike or dignified way. I was once the victim rather than the victor when it broke; it bruised everything on the front part of my body when the motor burned out and the tread siezed. There was an obvious tendency for the guys there to abuse the things the first time they showed weakness. Eventually, the management—rather than investing in new ones—began roping them off several days a week. I expected to see someone with a dry sense of humor attach an ON STRIKE sign, but that never materialized. The humidity in the gym made the printing run when I sneaked one into my locker to plant when everyone left.)

Our initial tendency is to discourage treadmill use. If you want to run, dress accordingly, get a good pair of running shoes, and go outside and run. We say that because we both enjoy running and because a treadmill can seem like an exercise in self-induced frustration. At least with the exercise cycle, you can keep your hands unoccupied and do something else at the same time.

There are, however, some very interesting treadmills on the market today. Some of them now feature monitoring devices that you can attach to yourself to get instant readouts, much like the instrument panel of a car. Many of the newer treadmills are also much more quiet when in operation than the old models.

Again, as with anything you buy, there are various levels of quality—and quality tends to increase with price. Unless you are very wealthy or unless you plan to make extensive use of your treadmill (and take meticulous care of it), we'd have to advise against buying one. By putting a mat down on your floor, you can run in place and get as much benefit. Or, as already mentioned, you can go outside and run. Before buying one or even thinking seriously about such a purchase, put on your running shorts and shoes and make the rounds of the stores that sell them, trying each one out for about fifteen minutes.

If you really want to use a treadmill on a regular basis, get a membership in your local health spa and use theirs, where you'll get to use all the other equipment and facilities along with it. In the long run (no pun), we think you'll be better served. Let the health spa pay for the repairs when you decide to try to break their treadmill.

WEIGHTS

Yes and no.

Talk about oversimplification, huh?

There was a period in the history of America, sometime back in the forgotten age of movies like "Muscle Beach Party Goes Bananas," when American males wanted some very basic things from life: A chopped and channeled roadster with wide tires and a rumbleseat large enough for a surfboard, a beach where the waves came in big and brazen all day, a beach that went on forever, and a set of muscles so big they could strut up and down that beach, looking at those waves, while golden girls looked at them and other guys stayed out of their way. Every Saturday night they could take the car to the dragstrip and make a trophy run. Ah, the simple days of youth.

That was the dream, see? Both of us, however, grew up in the Northeast, so we were three thousand miles removed from that scene, although every kid in America was very much in tune with it. With Beach Boys records on the AM radio and on "American Bandstand," the dream was hard to escape. The image has permeated American advertising ever since.

Some of the guys in those days became obsessed with their muscles. There was not an overabundance of health spas, however, so they sent away to places like York Barbell for sets of weights that the local postman got hernias delivering, or they made their own: they bought two buckets, a metal bar, and a bag of cement, and poured cement into one bucket, stuck the end of the bar into it, let it set, then poured the concrete into the other bucket, and pushed the free end of the bar into that bucket and, *voila!*, a set of weights. There was much huffing and puffing as they did their daily workouts, and much time standing in front of a mirror exploring for new-grown muscles. Unfortunately, the only things that grew with regularity and certainty on teenagers in those days were pimples.

Some of those kids persisted in their quest for the mighty muscle, and they are now seen strutting their stuff in the pages of the muscleman magazines that they used to hide under their mattresses. Muscle-building has even progressed to the point where it is becoming a craze among women, as you can't help but notice if you've read any of the national magazines within the year 1980.

Our main concern is building fitness and slimness instead of building bulk. Most weight sets are designed for bulking muscles. One begins at a certain level, and as progress is made, just continues to add weights, his or her level of strength being accommodated by the fact that you can come up with all types of weight combinations with your set.

As we've already indicated, your concentration should be with a multitude of repetitions with smaller weights. Few repetitions of a weight exercise with heavy weights will bulk; many repetitions of a weight exercise with light weights will slim.

Therefore, you could do with a partial set of weights if you've got your heart set on lifting weights. Most places, unfortunately, don't sell weight sets small enough to meet your needs. You'll end up with a lot of weights that you'll never use if you purchase the conventional package. You can, however, attempt to purchase pieces that you'll need. Or, better still, make a round of the garage and yard sales. You'll frequently be able to find a partial weight set that's seen better days (or sometimes, a weight set that's hardly been used) for a few dollars. Once you drag it home, you can use the larger weights for all sorts of things: doorstops, impressive paperweights, anchors for your dog's leash so it doesn't leave the yard...whatever. Then you can cull out the smaller weights and use them as a part of your daily exercise routine, concentrating on many reps.

Or, you can buy two sixty-four ounce bottles of liquid laundry detergent like we did, do your reps with those, and when you graduate to the gallon size, you can use the sixty-four ounce bottles to do your wash for the next month or two.

ROWING MACHINES

Rowing machines were very common forms of gym exercise apparatus at one point in history. They eventually gave way to other, less-cumbersome forms of equipment, and are now totally submerged (couldn't resist that one) under the Universal and Nautilus type equipment that combines many machines in one mother unit.

This is unfortunate, because rowing machines (although, as stated, cumbersome) are great devices for both building upper and lower body strength and tone, and for building the cardiovascular system.

The most common forms of exercise we think of when we think of aerobic exercise include running, jump rope and bicycling—exercises that provide continuous, low-level stress to build the body systems. They are all, however, oriented toward the lower body, primarily the legs. Swimming comes closest to allowing for equal use of arms and legs, but getting the use of a pool on a regular basis can be more of a nuisance than it's worth. As a result, people who are perfectly fit and who are beautiful examples of cardiovascular development often have underdeveloped upper-body strength. Runners are notorious for this.

The rowing machine can build upper-body strength and cardiovascular endurance if it is done correctly, i.e., beginning with a modest program and building as you become more and more fit. It must, like running, be done so as to stress but not strain the muscles. And it must be done on a regular program (at least three to four times a week) if it is to be beneficial.

A rowing machine, for those with space to use it and money to afford it, would probably be preferable to many of the other apparatus available. It is one of the only good aerobic/upper-body developers that cannot be done better outside...unless you wish to tow an actual boat or scull to the local river three or four times a week.

OTHER EQUIPMENT

With the marked influx of people exercising and working to become fit in the United States, the famed American ingenuity is again coming to the fore. We are seeing some very creative equipment and gadgets coming off the drawingboards and onto the advertising pages of magazines.

There is a jump rope that compacts into a small wand for easy transportation and that, when in use, squares the middle of the rope so that there is no mid-point bulge to wack against the ceiling if you jump rope indoors. Ingenious.

And there's the trampoline-like thing that is not a trampoline, but can serve as an indoor jogging pad. When not in use, it looks like a huge footstool. We're not fond of the fabric that covers it, as it looks like it would be more at home in a sultan's tent, but the idea is sound, even if no one bothered to figure out that you'd have to increase the height of the average ceiling if you were six feet and tried to use it. Perhaps it would be good for changing hard-to-reach lightbulbs or for dusting high corners.

Although we have not yet had an opportunity to try it out, there is apparently a home-size version of the exercise complex (similar to Nautilus and Universal) used in gyms. The home-size outfits apparently compact into a corner and offer all sorts of workout possibilities.

Some of the solutions to exercising at home are clever and many of them are reasonably priced. It is still our contention, however, that the best exercises are the most simple and those using the least apparatus. We can't help being impressed by some of the equipment, and if we had a closet in which to store it, we'd probably start a collection. Who knows? On a chilly, rainy winter Saturday afternoon, one's bent does sometimes turn to bizarre forms of amusement.

IN CONCLUSION

The amount of exercise equipment that we own is modest. It does not, in fact, go beyond what's outlined in the Bucket Brigade. We both have ten-speed bicycles as it's hard to pack a picnic lunch on an exercise cycle and stop along the way to lie under a tree and enjoy the lunch. This is not to say that exercise equipment cannot be a valuable exercising aid to you. We just like to keep our exercising indoors a bit less complicated.

With the warm-up exercises we've outlined, the Bucket Brigade and the ten minute sequence, we feel you're equipped with a basic arsenal of exercises. There are many more sequences we could present, and many variations, and many other strength and fitness builders. We'll save those for *Advanced Indoor Exercises*, however. Become familiar and intimate with the exercises here, make them a part of your daily life, and then either expand your exercising to the outdoors when weather permits, or stick with us for the next phase of indoor exercising.

If we can leave you with a few thoughts from this book, let them be these:

1. Begin an exercise program slowly and gently.

2. Exercise regularly once you begin.

3. Be patient; changes in your level of fitness and your body come gradually, and do not blossom fully-formed overnight. Keep your journal and you'll find that, like watching children grow, you don't notice it when you see them every day, but go away from them a few months and, when you check back, you'll be amazed at the changes.

4. Regularly elevate your goals as you raise your base through regular exercise. And keep your machine well-tuned and ready for a more thorough enjoyment of life.

Appendices

APPENDIX I
PROGRESSION AND MEASUREMENT TABLE

Before you begin your exercise program, you should measure yourself carefully. Periodically, you should take new measurements, always recording them faithfully.

Using the information provided in this book, you can devise an exercise program that is uniquely yours. Record the exercises you want to use on the chart that follows, and stick to them for ten consecutive sessions. Then remeasure yourself. If, after those ten sessions, you wish to add more exercises, do so if you feel that they will not strain you.

Once you begin your revised program, continue doing the same exercises for at least another ten sessions before measuring yourself again. This will enable you to see improvement if you're being faithful to the program by doing it a minimum of three times per week.

Your program should include six to ten exercises (not including warm-ups). Remember, if you begin by doing the least number of exercises the fewest possible times, you'll have plenty of room for improvement...and you will improve. Don't start too ambitiously and burn yourself out after three sessions. Be faithful to your exercise schedule, and to recording your progress in your journal (see Appendix II). Your progress will be easily followed and well-documented.

A sample Progression and Measurement Table follows. We've also provided a filled-in sample following the blank table. We invite you to make Xerox copies of the blank table and hang your current program up on the refrigerator door or some other place that will remind you of your program and that will also allow you easy access. When you are finished with your sessions on that sheet, save it in a loose-leaf binder. It's fun to consult your old programs periodically, both to see your increase in exercises, and to see your improvement in measurements.

PROGRESSION & MEASUREMENT CHART

DATE _____ MEASUREMENTS		EXERCISES CODE DESCRIPTION	reps / date	
UNDERARM **1** R.____ L.____	**1**		/	/
CHEST **2** _____	**2**		/	/
WAIST **3** _____	**3**		/	/
STOMACH **4** _____	**4**		/	/
HIPS **5** _____	**5**		/	/
THIGHS **6** R.____ L.____	**6**		/	/
CALVES **7** R.____ L.____	**7**		/	/
ANLKES **8** R.____ L.____	**8**		/	/
UPPER ARMS **9** R.____ L.____	**9**		/	/
WT _____ LBS.	**10**		/	/
HT. _____	**11**		/	/

PROGRESSION & MEASUREMENT CHART CONT.

								DATE _____
								MEASUREMENTS
								UNDERARM 1 R._____ L._____
								CHEST 2_____
								WAIST 3_____
								STOMACH 4_____
								HIPS 5_____
								THIGHS 6 R._____ L._____
								CALVES 7 R._____ L._____
								ANKLES 8 R._____ L._____
								UPPER ARMS 9 R._____ L._____
								WT._____ LBS.
								HT. _____

PROGRESSION & MEASUREMENT CHART

DATE 16 Nov. 80		EXERCISES		reps / date	
MEASUREMENTS		CODE	DESCRIPTION		
1 UNDERARM 40"	1	1-I	Hang Loose	4/16	4/17
2 CHEST 40"	2	1-II	Pull Leg	5/	5/
3 WAIST 32"	3	1-III	Cat	1/	1/
4 STOMACH 32"	4	1-IV	Twist	10/	10/
5 HIPS 37"	5	1-V	Rocking Chair	1/	—/
6 R. 22½" L. 22" THIGHS	6	1-VI	Bob	9/	6/
7 R. 15½" L. 15" CALVES	7	1-VII	Running	1/	1/
8 R. 9½" L. 9½" ANLKES	8	1-VIII	Jumping Jacks	10/	10/
9 R. 10" L. 10" UPPER ARMS	9	1-IX	Hand Clap	6/	4/
WT 165 LBS.	10	1-X	Circles	10/	7/
HT. 5'11 ¾"	11	1-+	Hot Shower	10/	10/

PROGRESSION & MEASUREMENT CHART CONT.

NOVEMBER

/18	5/19	4/20	5/21	/22	4/23	5/24	DATE **24 NOV. 80** MEASUREMENTS
— /	5 /	4 /	5 /	— /	4 /	5 /	UNDERARM 1 __40"__
— /	5 /	5 /	5 /	— /	4 /	4 /	CHEST 2 __40"__
— /	1 /	2 /	1 /	— /	1 /	2 /	WAIST 3 __32"__
— /	10 /	10 /	10 /	— /	5 /	5 /	STOMACH 4 __32"__
— /	1 /	1 /	— /	— /	— /	1 /	HIPS 5 __37__
— /	10 /	6 /	10 /	— /	— /	3 /	THIGHS 6 R. 22½ L. 22
— /	2 /	1 /	1 /	— /	2 /	2 /	CALVES 7 R. 15½ L. 15
— /	10 /	10 /	10 /	— /	5 /	5 /	ANKLES 8 R. 9½ L. 9½
— /	6 /	4 /	6 /	— /	2 /	3 /	UPPER ARMS 9 R. 10 L. 10
— /	10 /	7 /	10 /	— /	5 /	5 /	WT. __164__ LBS.
10 /	10 /	10 /	10 /	10 /	15 /	15 /	HT. __5' 11 ¾"__

APPENDIX II
WEEKLY JOURNAL

We read a lot in history books about "recorded history." Without some of an historical sense being recorded, we'd have no history. In other words, the existence of this earth is divided into two unequal parts: prehistoric times and (apparently) historic times.

The prehistoric are a lot longer than the historic times, because prehistoric times go all the way back to the creation of the earth. Archaeologists uncovering fossils of dinosaurs does not count as finding historical evidence; it apparently takes someone writing something down to constitute the real thing.

No one knows for sure who first thought to write something down. It was probably something of little importance at the time; perhaps a chip of rock in a cave that has some cryptic marks etched upon it: quart of goat's milk, loaf of bread, side of dinosaur.

Whatever the historical (or prehistorical) particulars, we do know one very important thing: Most of the books from the Alexandria library of ancient times have been lost forever, destroyed by raiding illiterates, while the trash dumps of long-gone civilizations continue to provide grist for the archaeologists' learned papers. Castles and great civilizations crumble and leave nothing, but the dumping areas of the common people read like a book. What lessons does that teach us?

1. Don't make fun of recycling engineers (dump pickers).

2. Watch what you discard in your trash, as archeologists snooping around dump sites two thousand years in the future may learn things about you you'd rather leave covered at the landfill.

3. Little scraps of information have lasting value.

Our concern here is with the latter piece of knowledge. We've already provided you with a recording tool for your specific exercises and exercise sessions (see Appendix I), which also includes an on-going review of your measurements. But that's all pretty technical and cold. Exercise is something that is very much a human activity. And human beings, being thinking creatures, have thoughts and feelings about the things they do. We have provided, on the pages following, a means of keeping a record of your very human responses to your exercising program. It is a simple journal. Very similar to a diary. You can merely fill in the month and the day of the month and then jot down the number of minutes you

Name: Dynamic Cycle (model DC 1)

Manufactured by:

Walton Manufacturing Company
106 Regal Row
Dallas, Texas 75247
(214) 637-2500

Price: $339.50

Description: Non-electric. Pedaling activates mechanically balanced unit. Foot straps, large padded seat and chromed handlebar heights are adjustable. Chrome-plated steel frame with vinyl-coated metal panels with Danish walnut wood-grain finish. Chain drive mechanism with pre-lubricated oilite or ball bearings at all movements. Features 2½ to 1 reduction from pedal revolution to handlebar and seat movement. Balanced steel flywheel maintains automatic action of pedals, handlebar and seat movements without a mechanical resistance control. Weighs seventy pounds.

Name: ErgoMetric Exerciser (model EX 2)

Manufactured by:

Schwinn Bicycle Company
1856 North Kostner Avenue
Chicago, Illinois 60639

Price: $683.00

Description: A stationary bicycle ergometer which permits a closely controlled, measured and repeatable cycling program. When pedaling, with the resistance control at one of eleven settings, energy expenditure remains relatively constant over a wide range of pedal speeds (fifty to ninety rpms). Thus, both the program and the rider's reaction to the program can be charted. A program chart is part of the console unit which can be used to record the length of time riding, the resistance load and the rpms. Instrument panel includes timer, odometer, speedometer and push-button activated pedal resistance control with dial settings. Dynamometer tested and rated. Solid state electronic regulation. Weighs seventy-three pounds.

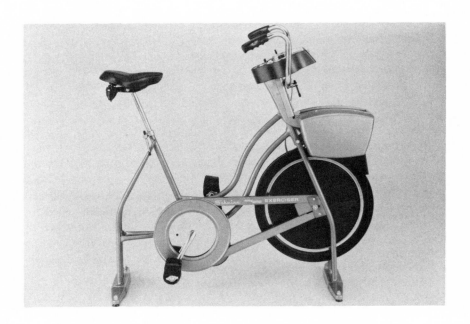

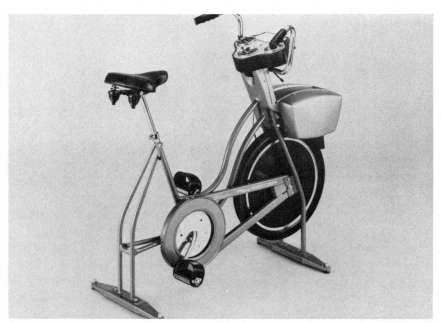

The ErgoMetric Exerciser by Schwinn features eleven different settings, with a pedal speed range of from fifty to ninety rpms.

Name: Europa 602

Manufactured by:

Vitamaster
455 Smith Street
Brooklyn, New York 11231
(212) 858-0505

Price: Available upon request

Description: Vitamaster offers a staggering array of exercise cycles—something for every taste and/or need. The Europa 602 is a sophisticated model manufactured with 1" to 1½" welded steel tube frame, dual steel chain guard, ball bearing pedals, extra wide front and rear legs, and equipped with cast aluminum weighted flywheel, speedometer/odometer, instant quick-lock handlebar adjustment, efficient, convenient caliper tension control. Chrome fender, thirty-minute bell ringing timer, conveniently located instrument panel, two-position pedal straps for forward and backward exercise and a super comfort chrome contour seat with removable padded seat cover. Weighs sixty pounds.

Name: Exercise Bike

Manufactured by:

Marcy Gym Equipment Company
2801 West Mission Road
Alhambra, California 91803
(213) 570-1222

Price: $475.00

Description: Designed for programs in which an accurate measurement of the workload being performed is desired. Features an odometer, speedometer, sixty-minute timer and a unique indicator which gauges braking force and the resulting muscle taxation. Precision machined 18 kg. flywheel for even resistance. Disc type brakes for rugged durability. Seat and handlebar are easily adjusted. Stores compactly. Requires 1½' x 3' of floor space.

Name: Exercise Slimmer (model MCA 10)

Manufactured by:

Merchants Corporation of America
14004 Anson Avenue
Santa Fe Springs, California 90670
(213) 802-1785

Price: $129.99

Description: Constructed with 1½" tubular steel. Speedometer and odometer. Full chain guard in high-impact polyurethane construction. Easy adjustable handlebar and seat. Minimum assembly; assembly wrench included. Primarily designed for women and children.

Name: Exercycle Executive

Manufactured by:

The Exercycle Corporation
667 Providence Street
Woonsocket, Rhode Island 02895

Price: Available upon request

Description: Two speeds (sixty and ninety pedal rpm), weight adjustment and ½-hp motor. Also has available the PEP (Personal Exercise Planner) with a stand, seat cushion and casters, all of which are available as accessories. This is the most popular of the Exercycle models.

Name: Exercycle Senior

Manufactured by:

The Exercycle Corporation
667 Providence Street
Woonsocket, Rhode Island 02895

Price: Available upon request

Description: Incorporates all the features of the Executive model, but is geared to a slower speed (thirty and forty-five pedal rpm). The length of each pedal crank can be adjusted for those with special needs.

Name: Exercycle Therapeutic

Manufactured by:

The Exercycle Corporation
667 Providence Street
Woonsocket, Rhode Island 02895

Price: Available upon request

Description: Incorporates all the features of the Executive model, including casters and seat cushion, but offers a fully variable speed motor which enables the pedal speed to be varied from zero to ninety rpm. The length of the pedal crank can be adjusted for those with special needs. This machine is especially suited for institutional and family use where a wide variety of physical capabilities need to be accommodated.

Name: The Explorer (model 455)

Manufactured by:

Walton Manufacturing Company
106 Regal Row
Dallas, Texas 75247
(214) 637-2500

Price: $219.50

Description: Sturdy welded frame constructed of one-inch diameter steel tubing. Heavy spoke rim with 20" x 1.75 tire covered with royal brown ABS discs. Twin chrome handlebars adjust for near or far reach without tools. Chain drive and positive finger tip tension control for smooth pedaling resistance. Speedometer with resettable odometer, thirty minute mechanical timer, set in convenient-to-reach console. Weighs sixty pounds.

Name: Flywheel Exercise Cycle (model MCA 14)

Manufactured by:

Merchants Corporation of America
14004 Anson Avenue
Santa Fe Springs, California 90670
(213) 802-1785

Price: $199.99

Description: Steel exercise bike, complete 1¾" tubular steel construction. Compact yet sturdy. Quick adjustment handlebar and seat stem for added comfort. Features seven tension settings utilized with handle gear. Complete with odometer, speedometer, timer and stirrups. Minimum assembly; comes with assembly wrench.

Name: Health Bike (model 012)

Manufactured by:

Battle Creek Equipment
307 West Jackson Street
Battle Creek, Michigan 49016
(616) 962-6181

Price: $169.00

Description: A speedometer records your speed and distance; a control knob allows you to increase resistance, requiring a more vigorous uphill push, and you can also pedal backwards to more fully develop leg muscles. Welded steel frame construction. Also features odometer and easy-adjust seat. Weighs thirty-five pounds.

Name: Matador Bike (model 411)

Manufactured by:

Walton Manufacturing Company
106 Regal Row
Dallas, Texas 75247
(214) 637-2500

Price: $159.50

Description: Tubular steel frame construction with one-inch diameter tubing and solid steel crossbars. Quick adjustment clamp for seat height. Handlebar easily lowered when necessary for storage and shipping. Chain drive. Heavy spoked rim and 20" x 1.75 tire. Fingertip control for adjusting pedaling tension. Speedometer and odometer. Weighs forty pounds.

Name: Monark Number 862

Manufactured by:

Dynamics Health Equipment Manufacturing Company
1538 College Avenue
South Houston, Texas 77587
(713) 946-5734

Price: Available upon request

Description: Features brake resistance shown on console scale (Newton-meter), plus a timer. Easily-adjustable saddle and handlebars, speedometer and odometer. Neatly collapsible for easy storage. Weighs thirty-three kilograms.

Name: Monark Number 867

Manufactured by:

Dynamic Health Equipment Manufacturing Company
1538 College Avenue
South Houston, Texas 77587
(713) 946-5734

Price: Available upon request

Description: A heavy-duty unit for excessive use in clubs, spas and schools. Seven tension adjustments. Speedometer and odometer. Large, well-balanced flywheel for smooth action. Easily adjustable saddle. Weighs twenty-two kilograms.

Name: Monark Number 872

Manufactured by:

Dynamic Health Equipment Manufacturing Company
1538 College Avenue
South Houston, Texas 77587
(713) 946-5734

Price: Available upon request

Description: Very simplified version of the exercise bicycle. Variable pedal resistance. Easily adjustable saddle and handlebars, speedometer and odometer. Weighs merely twenty-two kilograms.

Name: Regalcycle (model 014)

Manufactured by:

Battle Creek Equipment
307 West Jackson Street
Battle Creek, Michigan 49016
(616) 962-6181

Price: $789.00

Description: A manual cycling exerciser designed expressly for use in health clubs, salons and professional exercise establishments, but can also be purchased for the home. Weighs eighty-three pounds.

Name: Speed Bike (model 400)

Manufactured by:

Walton Manufacturing Company
106 Regal Row
Dallas, Texas 75247
(214) 637-2500

Price: $179.50

Description: Heavy-duty one-inch square tubular steel frame with royal brown enameled finish. Chain drive. Heavy spoked rim and 20" x 1.75 tire. Fingertip control for adjusting pedaling tension. Speedometer and odometer to indicate speed and mileage. Adjustable seat and handlebar height with special handlebar feature for swimming exercises. Weighs forty-five pounds.

Name: Trimcycle (model 007)

Manufactured by:

Battle Creek Equipment
307 West Jackson Street

Battle Creek, Michigan 49016

(616) 962-6181

Price: $769.00

Description: Two-speed motorized action guides the user through movements of rowing, riding, swimming and cycling. Locking coasters provide easy mobility. Can be operated manually, and the speed can be adjusted for a light or vigorous workout.

Name: Tunturi Ergometer

Distributed by:

Amerec Corporation

Post Office Box 3825

Bellevue, Washington 98009

(206) 643-1000

Price: Available upon request

Description: A continuous control for pedaling resistance, speedometer and odometer timer, fast adjustment of handlebar and seat height. Other devices from Tunturi can be attached. A tape meter indicates the crank movement and, at fifty and sixty rpm, the pedaling effect. Welded body of steel tubes. Low center of gravity and consequently, excellent stability.

Treadmills

Name: Contour Jogger (model 011)

Manufactured by:

Battle Creek Equipment

307 West Jackson Street

Battle Creek, Michigan 49016

(616) 962-6181

Price: $359.00

Description: A patented design that positions hard-maple rollers in a gentle arc under the tread belt. You start off on a level track, then progress up the curve as the tread moves smoothly under your feet. A pedometer registers the distance you run during each workout. The gentle slope requires extra effort, resulting in a more invigorating exercise session. Unit is forty-nine and one-half inches long, twenty inches wide and forty-five inches high, and weighs forty-nine pounds.

Name: Dyna-Pace

Manufactured by:
Dynamic Health Equipment Manufacturing Company
1538 College Avenue
South Houston, Texas 77587
(713) 946-5734

Price: Available upon request

Description: Heavy welded steel frame, ball-bearing roller bed, endless molded tread, sound-deadening aluminum rollers, dynamic pacing brake (½ to 25 mph governed speed range), fingertip speed control, perfect balance, fold-down handle for storage on end, transportation casters, high-inertia roller system, variable incline grade elevation (two to fourteen percent), speedometer, tripometer. Weighs one hundred thirty-five pounds in shipping.

Name: Health Walker (model 004)

Manufactured by:
Battle Creek Equipment
307 West Jackson Street
Battle Creek, Michigan 49016
(616) 962-6181

Price: $469.00

Description: Adjustable side rails for added stability. Includes a pedometer to measure distance traveled. Inclined for more vigorous exercising. Features support strap and stabilizer bar. Weighs seventy-four pounds.

Name: Marcy Treadmill Number 2010

Manufactured by:
Marcy Gym Equipment Company
2801 West Mission Road
Alhambra, California 91803
(213) 570-1222

Price: $495.00

Description: Designed for institutional use, the treadmill features all steel welded construction. Its patented design attempts to duplicate the running motion of jogging outdoors. The inclined running surface with raised end portion allows the user to vary the speed by where the runner is positioned on the treadmill. The front portion provides a fast running action, while the rear of the unit is designed for walking speed. Offers the advantage of a motorized unit but with an affordable price and reputedly low maintenance. Extra-long running surface with twenty-one two-inch durable steel conveyor type rollers with sealed self-lubricating ball bearings and two four-inch flanged end rollers to help keep the belt centered. Features a speedometer/odometer, chrome handrails and foam-padded vinyl side panels.

Name: Marcy Treadmill Number 2011

Manufactured by:

Marcy Gym Equipment Company
2801 West Mission Road
Alhambra, California 91803
(213) 570-1222

Price: $675.00

Description: Features the same rugged construction of the Number 2010 model by Marcy, but is shorter (forty-four inches) with eighteen two-inch steel rollers and two four-inch flanged end rollers.

Name: The Olympian Jogger (model 655 SR)

Manufactured by:

Walton Manufacturing Company
106 Regal Row
Dallas, Texas 75247
(214) 637-2500

Price: $499.50

Description: Curved running surface for smooth, quiet self-pacing walking, jogging or running action. This non-electric unit has thirty steel rollers, each turning on two pre-lubricated ball bearings supported by walnut-look side panels. Belt guides keep extra wide running belt properly positioned. Welded steel frame supports chrome-plated steel front and side rails. Speedometer and resettable odometer housed in ABS console. Also has thirty-minute mechanical timer. New handlebar design. Weighs one hundred ten pounds.

Name: Pace-Setter 2001

Distributed by:

American Athletic Company

5302 Gulfton, Building Number 1
Houston, Texas 77081
(713) 667-9606
Toll free: 800-231-6652

Price: $595.00

Description: A standard treadmill forty-eight inches high and twenty-two inches wide with chrome handrails, a speedometer and odometer, full frame of all steel and a foam-padded naugahyde covering for the frame. Two-ply heavy-duty conveyer belt provides cushioned running surface that is concave to allow individual to walk, jog or run at his or her own pace. Features patented flanged end rolls to keep belt centered and thus eliminate wear.

Name: Runabout Jogger (model 644 SR)

Manufactured by:

Walton Manufacturing Company
106 Regal Row
Dallas, Texas 75247
(214) 637-2500

Price: $299.50

$279.50 (without side rails)

Description: Chrome-plated steel front rail and steel side rails that extend the length of the unit. Mechanical unit with all steel frame and dual belt guides. Heavy woven laced belt (fourteen inches wide) moves over plated steel rollers turning in oilite bearings. Adjustable knobs for belt tensioning and adjustable incline angle. Has speedometer and odometer. Sides are covered with vinyl-clad steel. Weighs sixty pounds.

Name: Treadmill Jogger (model 600 SR)

Manufactured by:

Walton Manufacturing Company
106 Regal Row
Dallas, Texas 75247
(214) 637-2500

Price: $399.50

Description: A non-electric unit with chrome-plated steel front rail and chrome-plated side rails. Heavy steel frame construction. Smooth-turning steel rollers revolve in oilite bearings.

Front and rear rollers are housed in ball bearings for a smoother action. Has 14" x 85" laced belt, treated for wear resistance and scuffing. Two adjustment knobs for precise tracking of belt in addition to incline angle for light or active resistance to belt. Unit features speedometer and resettable odometer. Weighs seventy pounds.

Name: Tredex

Manufactured by:

American Tredex Corporation
1450 Wabash Avenue
Post Office Box 1047
Terre Haute, Indiana 47808
(812) 238-2902
Toll free: 800-457-0771

Price: Available upon request

Description: An ultra-modern, sophisticated treadmill featuring solid state electronics and innovative engineering. The readout control panel resembles the control panel of a 747, and features a capacity for holding four modes of information constantly, a display of speed, distance and time, speed increase and decrease controls, and a heart rate monitoring unit and display that can be hooked up to the runner. Also features safety handles with a built-in emergency shut-off system. A no-stretch belt that travels across a silicone-impregnated birchwood surface for comfortable running.

Name: Walker-Jogger Deluxe (model J-35)

Manufactured by:

Vitamaster
455 Smith Street
Brooklyn, New York 11231
(212) 858-0505

Price: Available upon request

Description: The J-35 incorporates conveniently built-in instrument panel, reset speedometer/odometer (can be reset for each exercise session), bell ringing timer, eighteen hardwood rollers, three-inch special drive drum for more accurate speedometer/odometer calibration, heavy-duty endless reinforced rubber belt, two four-pound chrome cast iron flywheels, chrome adjustable front handle for smooth operation, level or uphill incline, chrome side rails adjustable for height, wood-grain formica finish and solid plywood frame. Weighs sixty-five pounds in shipping.

Weights

Name: Code-A-Wate

Manufactured by:

Banyan International Corporation
2118 East Interstate 20
Post Office Box 1779
Abilene, Texas 79604
(915) 677-1874

Prices: $5.50 to $49.30

Description: A complete system of physical therapy weights that are color-coded, Velcro closing, reinforced vinyl, nylon stitching. An excellent system for those who want to use weights to supplement their exercise program; nothing massive and gym-like.

Rowing Machines

Name: Adjustable Tension Rowing Maching (model MCA 1200)

Manufactured by:

Merchants Corporation of America
14004 Anson Avenue
Santa Fe Springs, California 90670
(213) 802-1785

Price: $199.99

Description: Constructed with one and one-half inch tubular chrome steel and one and one-fourth inch tubular painted steel. Interlocking chrome steel pins makes unit construction easy. Leather footstraps enables easy rowing exercise performance in a stabilized position while exercising. Casters allow the seat to flow easily and evenly with individual rowing. Independent tension controls allow for separate degrees of resistance in each rowing arm. Swivel handle grips cut down friction and fatigue and maximize fitness results.

Name: Dyna-Row 100

Manufactured by:

Dynamics Health Equipment Manufacturing Company
1538 College Avenue
South Houston, Texas 77587
(713) 946-5734

Price: Available upon request

Description: Chrome-plated steel frame, large contoured cushioned seat, dual hydraulic cylinders that adjust independently to control the dynamic rowing resistance, aluminum foot plate, large no-mar feet to prevent sliding and protect floors, nylon rollers under seat to insure a smooth ride, and designed to stand on end for compact, easy storage.

Name: Exerow II (model 001)

Manufactured by:

Battle Creek Equipment
307 West Jackson Street
Battle Creek, Michigan 49016
(616) 962-6181

Price: $999.00

Description: Perhaps the ultimate rowing machine, it is built to withstand institutional use with durable construction and strong, adjustable hydraulic resistance. As you pull the handlebars toward you, you push the foot pedals downward, stretching, flexing, bending and stimulating. Weighs seventy-four pounds.

Name: Ro-Trim (model 003)

Manufactured by:

Battle Creek Equipment
307 West Jackson Street
Battle Creek, Michigan 49016
(616) 962-6181

Price: $539.00

Description: A sturdy machine for rowing and bending exercises. Features adjustable resistance and sturdy construction. Basic, but one of the best forms of indoor equipment you can use. Weighs forty-five pounds, and is forty-six inches long, twenty-two inches wide and twenty-one inches high.

Name: Rower Exercise Cycle (model MCA 17)

Manufactured by:

Merchants Corporation of America

14004 Anson Avenue

Santa Fe Springs, California 90607

(213) 802-1785

Price: $229.99

Description: Features a dynometer and rowing action. Exercises both upper and lower parts of the body. Can be used for both pedaling and rowing....separately or together. Features separate tension controls, timer, speedometer, odometer and adjustment wrench. Comfortable, oversize seat.

Name: Tunturi Rowing Machine

Distributed by:

Amerec Corporation

Post Office Box 3825

Bellevue, Washington 98009

(206) 643-1000

Price: Available upon request

Description: Includes two hydraulic elements which efficiently simulate actual rowing. It is constructed to withstand heavy daily use. Features a continuous adjustment of braking resistance for each of the two oars, a sliding, anatomically designed seat as in competition rowing boats, and foot supports with adjustable straps, making the rowing machine suitable also for training the back and stomach muscles. Made from solid steel, chrome plated and painted. Insulated from the floor by plastic caps and is therefore silent, stable and safe. When not in use, it is stored vertically and thus takes up very little space. As optional equipment, there is a counter for checking the number of pulls.

Other Equipment

Name: Bullworker 3 (and Lady Bullworker)

Available: Sears Stores

Price: Men's $34.50—Ladies' $29.99

Description: Chrome-plated tubular steel with strong compressive steel spring inside; plastic grips, vinyl-covered steel cables, thirty-four and one-half inches long. Relies upon isometric

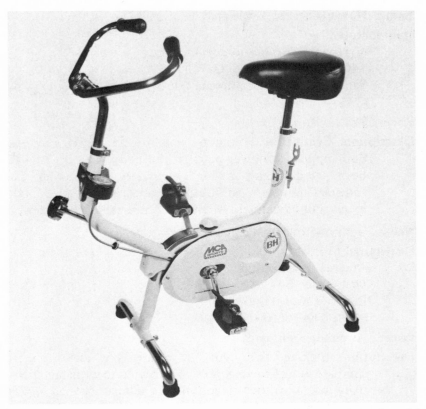

The MCA 17 is a combination of the rower machine and the exercise cycle and is excellent for exercising the upper and the lower body simultaneously.

contraction to help build and tone muscles. Very applicable for home use.

Name: Doorway Chinning Bar

Available: Sears Stores

Price: $9.99

Description: Chrome-plated steel bar, with stabilizing door clips, fits doorways twenty-five to thirty-two inches wide. Your basic chinning bar.

Name: Indoor Jogger

Manufactured by:

Dynamics Health Equipment Manufacturing Company
1538 College Avenue
South Houston, Texas 77587
(713) 946-5734

Price: Available upon request

Description: Six removable legs, molded spring cover, six-sided chromed steel frame for stability, cadmium plated, thirty-six spring suspension system engineered and tested for ultimate spring life, under warranty for one year for material and workmanship.

Name: Jogger's Rope

Manufactured by:

DB & K
18623 Santa Isadora
Fountain Valley, California 92708
(714) 963-5482

Price: $5.95 (plus $1.00 for postage and handling).

Description: Designed for indoor use, it swings "square" so you can jump indoors without hitting the ceiling. It comes with hollow walnut handles that snap together to form a storage case for the rope when not in use. The secret lies in a light-weight rope equipped with shaping weights.

Name: Jump-Rope

Available: Sears Stores

Price: Ball-Bearing Swivel Jump Rope $6.89
Lifeline Jump Rope $4.89
Swivel Jump Rope $2.89

Description: Variations on the basic stolen clothesline theme.

Name: Professional Total Gym

Manufactured by:

Total Medical Systems
7730 Clairemont Mesa Boulevard
San Diego, California 92111
(714) 560-5771

Price: $625.00

Description: Provides both osotonic and variable resistance that utilizes a percentage of one's own body weight as the workload. More than fifty specific exercises are possible on the apparatus. The frame is two inches by one inch, .083 rectangular heavy gauge, chrome-plated rectangular steel tubing; the ladder is one and one-fourth inches by one and one-fourth inches, .120 square steel tubing with solid 7/16" thick steel support hooks. Overall length is nine feet, width is three feet. Weighs one hundred fifty pounds in shipping.

Name: Push-Pull Muscle Developer

Available: Sears Stores

Price: $18.99

Description: Black, high-impact plastic. With handles attached, helps develop arms, back, leg muscles by resisting being pulled apart; with handles removed, pushing against it helps develop chest and shoulder muscles. Another isometric device. Dial adjusts length of travel, degree of difficulty. Compact and easy to store and transport in your gym bag.

Name: Sears Modular Home Gym

Available: Sears Stores

Price: $349.94 (does not include weights)

Description: A "complete" system that folds into a 10.3 square foot storage space when not in use; includes weight pulley assembly, lat bar, leg pulley assembly, preacher curl and neck developer. Certainly not the heavy-duty, long-lasting item, but, carefully taken care of, should last a good, long time for the casual user.

Name: Soloflex

Manufactured by:
The Wilson Design Group, Incorporated

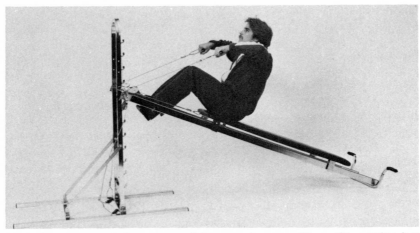

The Professional Total Gym concept brings together some 50 specific exercises into one relatively easy-to-use apparatus.

Hawthorn Farms Industrial Park
Hillsboro, Oregon 97123
800-547-8802

Price: $495.00

Description: Two dozen different exercise station variations in one based on progressive resistance. A series of intricately woven rubber rings, each resilient and reliable, provides the resistance. Takes up a surprisingly small amount of space. A whole gym in a corner.

Acknowledgments

The authors would like to thank certain people for their cooperation in making this book come together. Thanks to Jeff Reinking and David K. Madison Photography for studio work and to Sharon Rooney for endless hours of reading the book while it went together and after it was typeset. And to the following Northern California companies for their help in gathering information on indoor exercise apparatus: Advanced Fitness Equipment of Northern California of South San Francisco, Livingston Medical Products of Palo Alto, Los Gatos Equipment Center of Los Gatos, Palo Alto Orthopedic Company of Palo Alto, Corsi Joe Physical Fitness Equipment of Hayward and Rhea's Schwinn Cyclery of Palo Alto.

About the Authors

Richard Benyo is executive editor of *Runner's World Magazine* and editorial director of *Skier's World*. He has authored several other books, among them *Return to Running* and *Superspeedway*. A veteran of many marathons and ultramarathons, he does flexibility and strengthening exercises following his daily training runs. Skinny in high school, Benyo swelled to two hundred seven pounds before he turned thirty, but came down to one hundred fifty-five pounds following a resumption of a regular exercise program.

Rhonda Provost is a nurse anesthetist from Boston. Her profession gives her a healthy background in medicine and science. She has been living the type of life she advocates for as long as she can remember. She currently resides in Palo Alto, California, where she is a member of a local health spa, runs, and is an avid cyclist.

Recommended Reading

The following books, also available from Anderson World, can augment your exercise and fitness program. They are available from major bookstores or can be ordered directly from the publisher (1400 Stierlin Road, Mountain View, CA. 94043).

THE RUNNER'S WORLD YOGA BOOK by Jean Couch with Nell Weaver. An easy-to-follow guide to using the principles of yoga for stretching, strengthening, and toning the body, and a good book to graduate to after you've outgrown some of the exercise routines in *The Runner's World Indoor Exercise Book.* Spiral bound. $11.95

COMPLETE WOMEN'S WEIGHT TRAINING GUIDE by Edie Leen. Weight training for women has become a new trend in American fitness. Not so much to bulk muscles, but rather to properly tone them, women are embarking on weight programs both at gyms and in the privacy of their homes. $5.95

TOTAL WOMAN'S FITNESS GUIDE by Gail Shierman, Ph.D., and Christine Haycock, M.D. A good guide to choosing a fitness program that fits your needs, your goals, and your lifestyle, with special attention to what happens to a woman's body during physical activity. $4.95

THE COMPLETE DIET GUIDE edited by Hal Higdon. Optimal health is made more possible by using good nutrition. This book examines the athlete's diet in detail, with excellent information from doctors, coaches, trainers, and the athletes themselves. $4.95..

THE COMPLETE WOMAN RUNNER edited by the editors of *Runner's World.* Everything the woman contemplating taking up running as a viable exercise needs to know about the activity as a sport and as a lifestyle. $10.95.

RETURN TO RUNNING by Richard Benyo. The co-author of *The Runner's World Indoor Exercise Book* tells an inspiring story of a return to fitness following a decade of letting himself go to flab. Fun reading. $3.95.